The Alkaline Diet

The Elegant Recipes for Weight Loss, Healing and Detoxing

BY: Ivy Hope

Copyright © 2020 by Ivy Hope

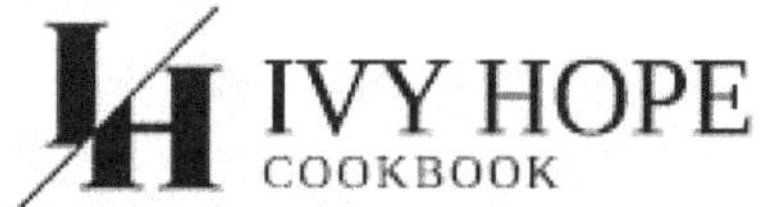

Copyright/License Page

Table of Contents

Introduction

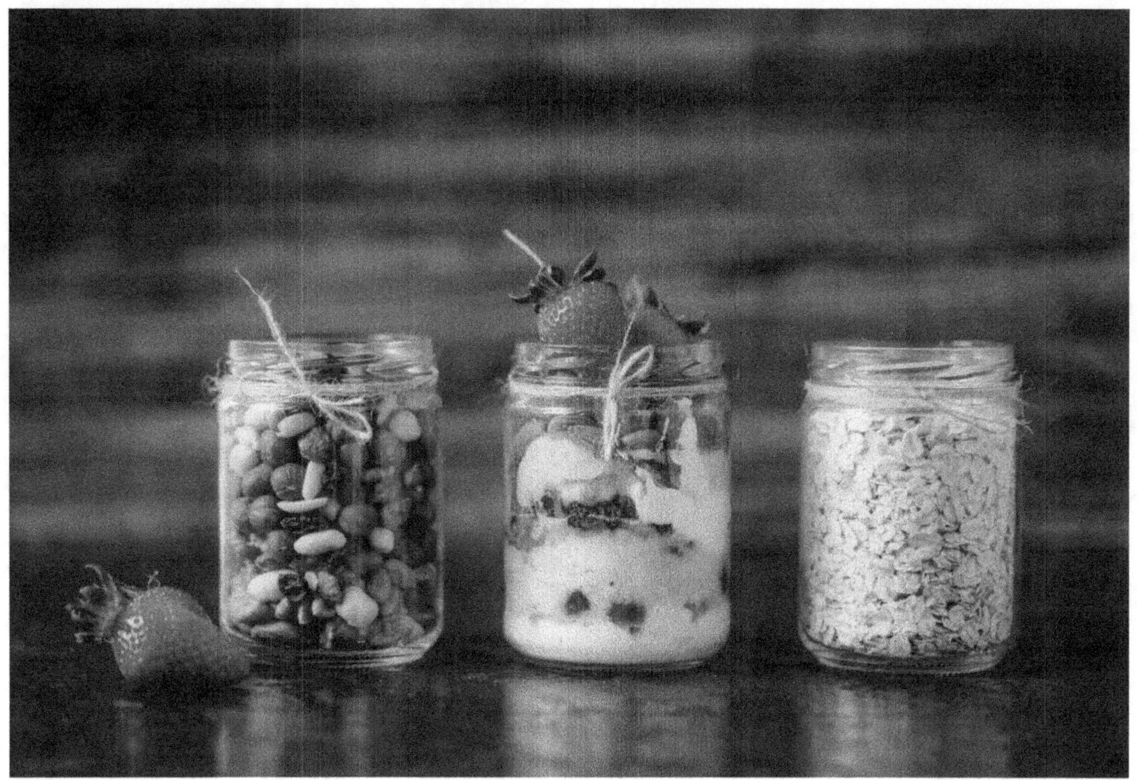

The human body is an amazing machine. All the systems inside the body were designed to work together to form a complete being capable of accomplishing many things. Human can walk, talk, think, and act. But the best performance depends on the human body working at the highest level at which it can possibly function. For this to be true, all the systems need to be balanced and healthy.

When there is an imbalance in one of the systems, that part of the body sends a message to the brain that says something is wrong. The stomach and digestive tract are one of the systems in the body, and when it is not in balance, it sends a message to the brain, letting the brain know something is not right.

Stomach imbalances can lead to low energy levels, poor digestion, and erratic mood swings. The stomach and the intestines have a major job to do for the body and it is important to keep them working well.

The stomach is the major component in the digestion of food that the body uses for energy. The stomach first secretes an acid that helps break down food, and the muscles move around to assist with the process. Then the food, which is now mostly processed and the nutrients gathered from it, is sent into the intestines for further processing and disposal. If the stomach cannot properly digest the food, it is unable to extract needed nutrients from that food. Then the stomach becomes off-balance.

But the alkaline diet is designed to avoid all those imbalance problems. Alkaline foods will battle against the acid in the stomach and make it easier for the stomach to digest foods. Acid does not come just from the stomach itself but also from various acidic foods that are consumed and must be digested. By avoiding acidic foods in favor of more alkaline foods, the stomach can return to its normal state of digestion and once again operate at top performance.

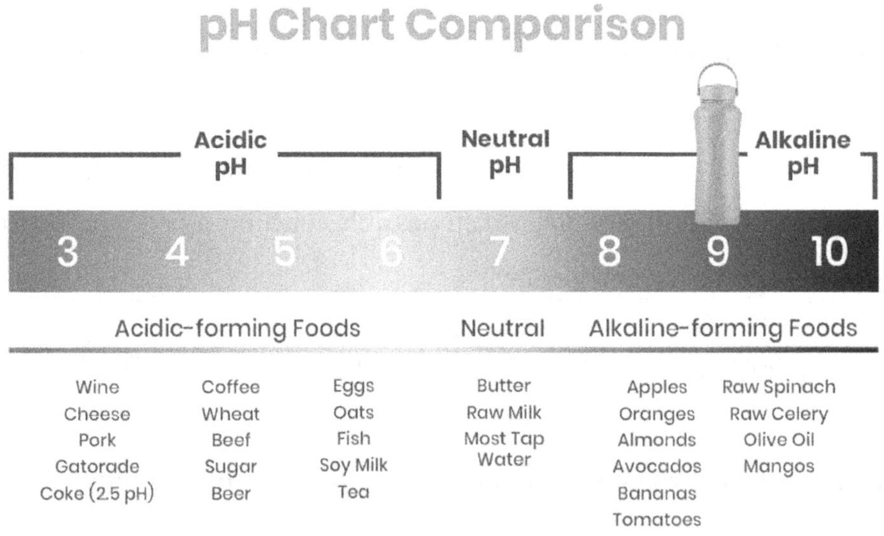

What is the Alkaline Diet?

The alkaline diet, or the alkaline ash diet, takes a whole new approach to what we consume. It does not consider the proportions or the nutritional composition of foods like other diets do. Instead, it considers the effects the different types of metabolic waste products after food has been digested and assimilated. The type of food determines the nature of its metabolic waste. Therefore, food containing acid compounds or acidic elements produces acidic waste, whereas alkaline foods produce alkaline metabolic waste. The experts who first suggested the idea of an alkaline diet for a healthier living say that acidic metabolic waste is harmful to bodily health as it can disrupt the optimal pH levels within the body which are essential to regulating enzyme function, hormone production, and other metabolic reactions. That is why the alkaline diet was proposed, it can help maintain the internal alkaline environment through the production of alkaline metabolic waste.

The alkaline diet is based on scientific research that studied the various effects of foods consumed on different organs in the body. They specifically focused on the stomach and the kidneys because the stomach digests the food and the kidneys are in charge of removing excess acid from the body through urine. It was found that certain food will raise the natural pH level in the body. pH is a measurement of a solution to find out how much hydrogen ion is in the solution. Hydrogen ions are a substance in the body that keeps the proteins in the body linked together in the shape they must stay in to be able to do their job in the body. Proteins play many important roles in the body. They carry messages to and from the brain. They help the body create antibodies to fight disease and infection. They provide support and structure for the cells and help carry vital nutrients to the cells. Hydrogen ions keep the protein cells linked together, so they can do their job. If the pH level of the body is too low, then the body has become acidic and the hydrogen ions are no longer strong enough to support the work of the proteins.

The alkaline diet helps keep the body at an even pH level to avoid the disruption of the work of the hydrogen ions and the proteins in the body.

When people eat, the body metabolizes the food and turns it into energy for the body to use. The alkaline diet specifically promotes the intake of alkaline type foods in order to keep the pH level of the body in a more alkaline, not acidic, state. The diet has a specific list of foods to eat and foods to avoid achieving this alkaline state.

The alkaline diet has been used for years by people who subscribe to and practice alternative forms of medicine. The diet offers smart eating choices that will balance out the pH level in the body and allow the body to return to the way it used to function back when the ancestors of modern man ate a similar diet and remained largely disease free.

Using the alkaline diet is an important first step toward a healthier lifestyle by promoting healthy bodily functions through a proper diet.

How Can You Lose Weight Naturally?

Highly acidic foods are, in most cases, very unhealthy and can often contribute to obesity. Acid-promoting foods affect the fat-burning capabilities of your body, while also affecting that you feel hungry more often. On the other hand, alkaline-promoting foods are considered anti-inflammatory. That gives you the chance to eat the right amount of calories and feel full after eating them. All this contributes to getting your weight in order and maintaining it.

Other health benefits of a balanced alkaline diet include anti-aging effects, such as your skin being more youthful and elastic. It also increases your energy levels and your mental alertness, while securing proper digestion and better sleep at night.

First things first, it is important to understand how acidic-forming foods negatively affect our bodies, which is mainly through the red blood cells. The red blood cells have a mechanism that enables them to stay away from each other. This is basically a negative charge that keeps them separate from one another. Increased acidity in the blood can mess up this mechanism by robbing the red blood cells of the negative charge. This will lead to the red blood cells clumping up together, which will limit the levels of oxygen that enters your cells. Increased acidity in your blood, therefore, can lead to the weakening and death of red blood cells.

Now, for the benefits of an alkaline diet:

Battles Fatigue

Too much acidity in your system decreases oxygen supply, which in turn decreases your cells' ability to repair and gather up nutrients. When your body lacks enough nutrients to give it energy, you will certainly feel weak. If you have been feeling tired and dazed through the day yet you had enough sleep, then you might need to check up on your acidity levels.

Boosts the immune system

An unbalance in pH lowers your body's ability to fight viruses and bacteria. There is a lack of oxygen in the system (which acidity causes, as explained above), viruses and bacteria flourish easily in the bloodstream. To eliminate the probability of diseases happening, alkalizing is essential.

Strengthens your bones

The more people age, the more the body uses up calcium, especially if you eat more acid-based foods. When we eat foods with high acidity, the body needs to balance the acid by dispensing calcium, magnesium and phosphorus. More than often, these minerals are taken from the bone stores, which can be a huge problem in the long run. But don't worry, with the alkaline diet, since you are not taking less of acid-forming foods, your body does not need to extract these minerals from your bones. In addition, you consume more of these minerals from the many alkaline foods high in these minerals.

A healthier body and weight loss

The alkaline diet provides a base for a rather healthy diet. First, the diet requires you to cut out/reduce alcohol, red meats, sugars, trans fats and processed foods, which will definitely help you with weight loss and offer you other numerous health benefits. Also, the diet requires you to increase your intake of fresh and healthy foods such as veggies and fruits and water, which boost your general health and increase your chances of losing weight.

Understanding pH

Now that you have a good grasp of the core concept of Alkaline diet, then let me explain the concept of "pH" levels.

A good understanding of pH levels is exceptionally crucial to comprehend further how Alkaline diet works.

So, generally speaking, pH is a component of our blood that is known as the "Potential of Hydrogen."

While assessing the level of pH in a liquid, it is possible to determine whether a liquid is alkaline, acidic or neutral.

Regarding humans, we usually measure the acidity or alkalinity of body fluids and tissue.

The measurement is done on a scale of 0-14 (refer to the picture above). The standard convention of reading the scale is as follows:

- The lower the pH value, the more acidic a solution is
- The higher the value goes, the more alkaline the solution is
- 7 is considered to be the neutral point on the scale

The pH level of our body usually stays at 7.4, which is deemed to be the safe point at which the body's mechanism works at optimal efficiency.

However, it has been deduced by researchers that a slight increase in the alkalinity level of pH tends to improve the overall health condition of the body significantly.

It should be noted though that the pH level of the body varies from one region to the next. For example, the stomach is generally regarded as naturally being the most acidic part of the body.

If the natural level of pH gets altered by even a slight amount, the body of human beings, as well as many other organisms, starts to react negatively.

A good example would be the recent increase of Carbon Di-Oxide disposition which led to a substantial slight decrease in the ocean's pH, where it went to 8.1 from 8.2. And a 0.1 change in pH, means various aquatic organisms and life forms have started to suffer.

This pH level is not only essential for plant growth but also forms part of the minerals in our food.

But every single organism has several means of defending the body from such changes. In the case of human beings, various minerals contribute by acting as a "buffer" to normalize the pH level of our body should it become more acidic!

Breakfast

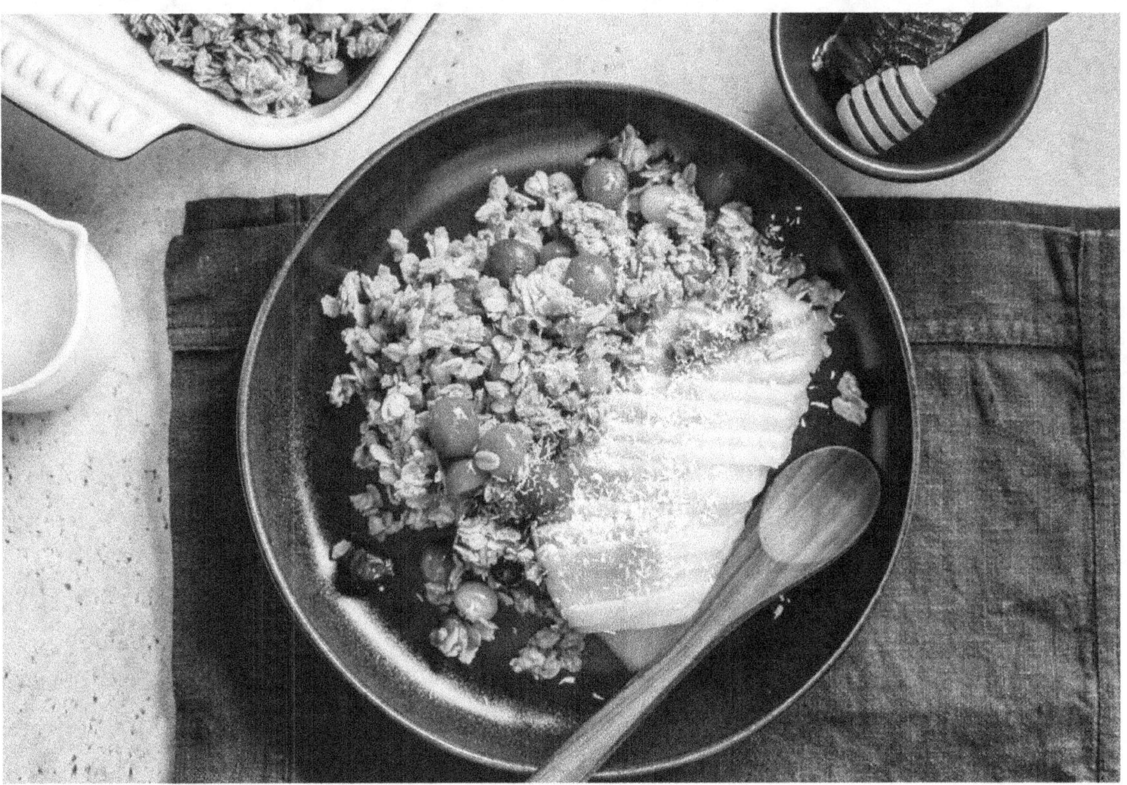

Hearty and delicious, the fiber-enriched bowl of rustic and hearty fare will keep the growling tummy at bay. While the ingredients may change from time to time, the result is a flavorful and delicious filling breakfast.

Chia and Almond Pudding

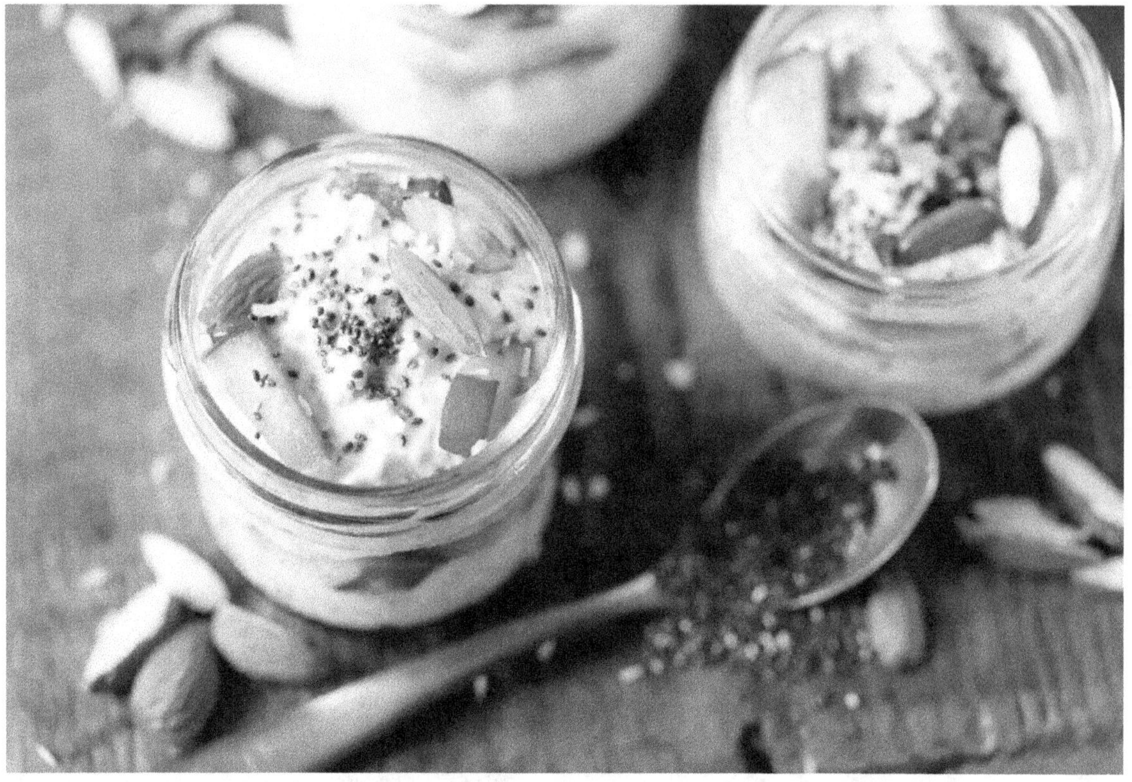

Chia Seed Pudding is a nice recipe for those of you who are on an alkaline diet. It is a great recipe with lots of nutritional value. It is also very low in fat. So, those of you who do not want to lose weight, you can eat as much of it as you want.

Cook time: 10 minutes

Servings: 3

Ingredients:

- 2 c. unsweetened almond milk
- ½ c. chia seeds
- 1 tsp. organic vanilla extract
- 1 tbsp. maple syrup
- ⅓ fresh strawberries, hulled and sliced
- 2 tbsp. almonds, sliced

Directions

In a large bowl, add the first four ingredients, extract and stir to combine well.

Refrigerate for about 3-4 hours, stirring occasionally.

Serve with the sliced strawberry and almond slice topping.

Amaranth Porridge

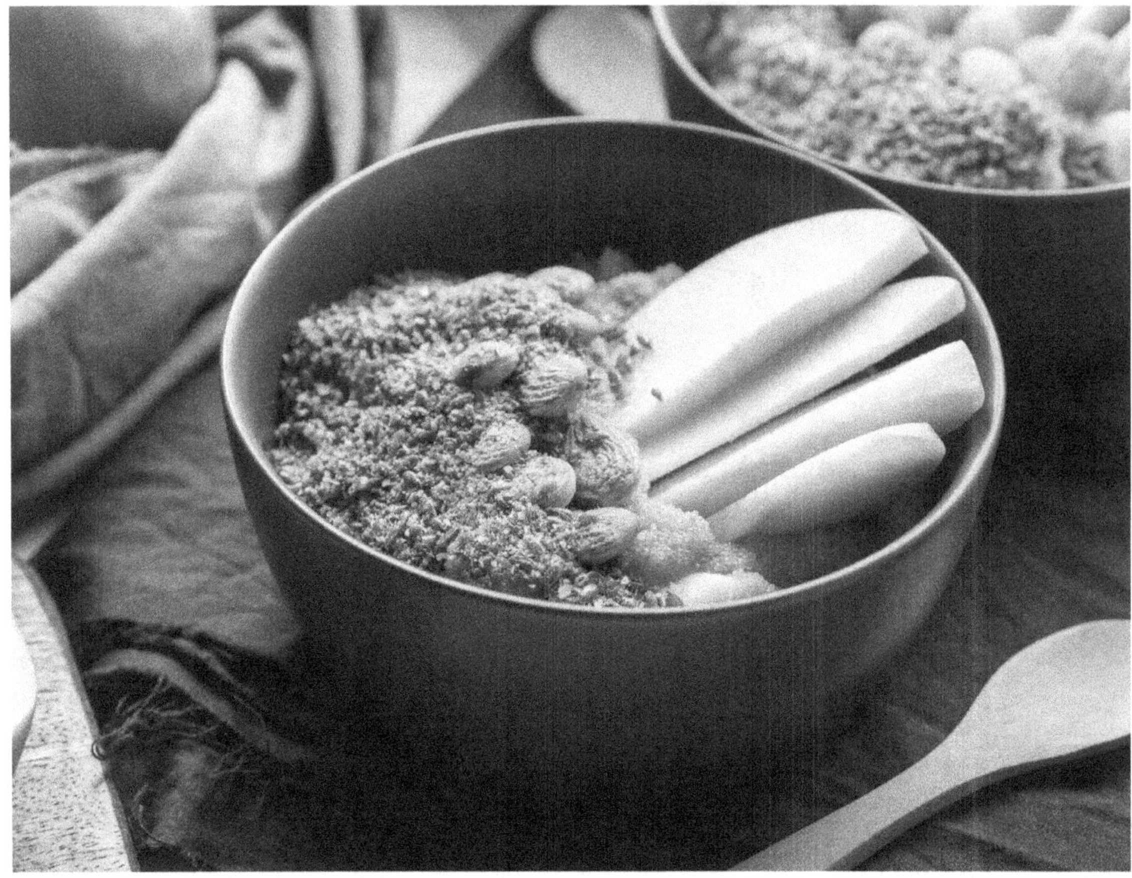

Amaranth Porridge is a very nutritious whole grain superfood. This gluten-free dish is best eaten soaked overnight and cooked in the morning.

Cook time: 35 minutes

Servings: 2

Ingredients:

- 2 c. almond milk
- 2 c. alkaline water
- 1 c. amaranth
- 2 tbsp. coconut oil
- 1 tbsp. ground cinnamon

Directions

Mix milk with water in a medium saucepan.

Bring the mixture to a boil.

Stir in amaranth then reduce the heat to low.

Cook on low simmer for 30 minutes with occasional stirring.

Turn off the heat. Stir in cinnamon and coconut oil.

Serve warm.

Zucchini Muffins

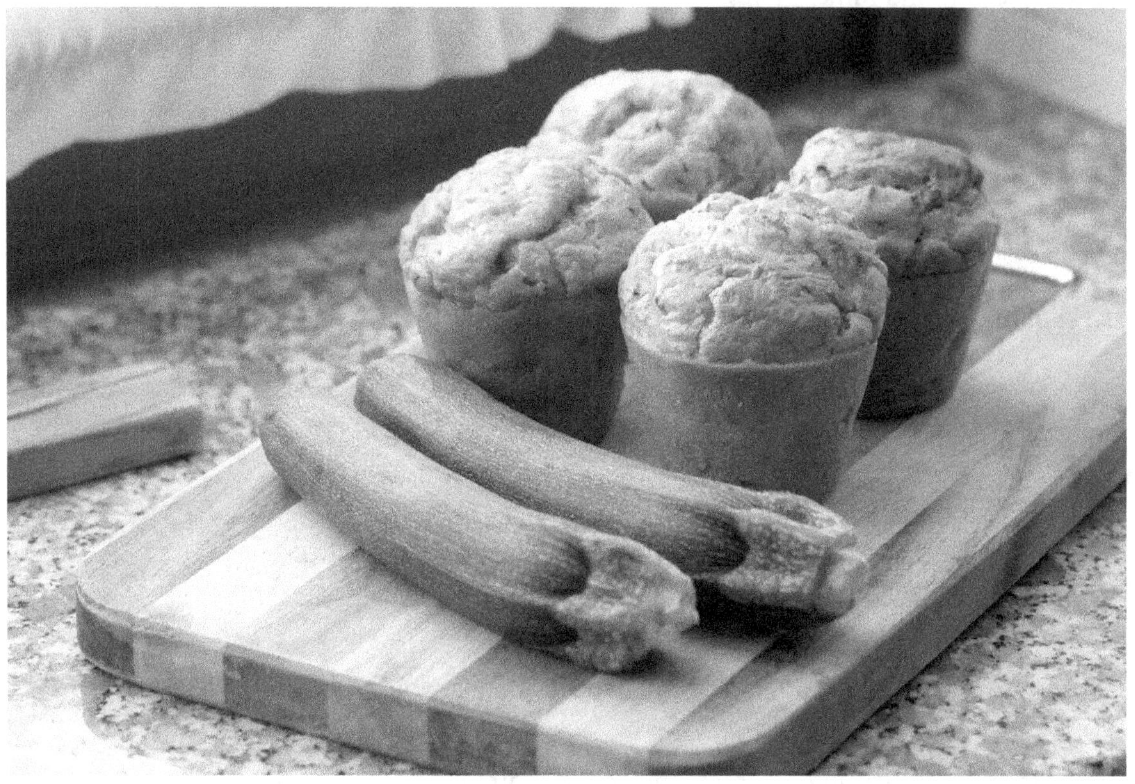

Zucchini Muffins are a healthy alternative to the typical starchy muffin. It is a delicious sweet vegetable bread that is packed with baked zucchini, vanilla, and flaxseed.

Cook time: 35 minutes

Servings: 16

Ingredients:

- 1 tbsp. ground flaxseed
- 3 tbsp. alkaline water
- ¼ c. almond butter
- 3 small-medium over-ripe bananas
- 2 small zucchinis, grated
- ½ c. almond milk
- 1 tsp. vanilla extract
- 2 c. almond flour
- 1 tbsp. baking powder
- 1 tsp. cinnamon
- ¼ tsp. sea salt

Optional add-ins:

- ¼ c. chocolate chips and/or walnuts

Directions

Set your oven to 375 degrees F. Grease a muffin tray with cooking spray.

Mix flaxseed with water in a bowl.

Mash bananas in a glass bowl and stir in all the remaining ingredients.

Mix well and divide the mixture into the muffin tray.

Bake for 25 minutes.

Millet Porridge

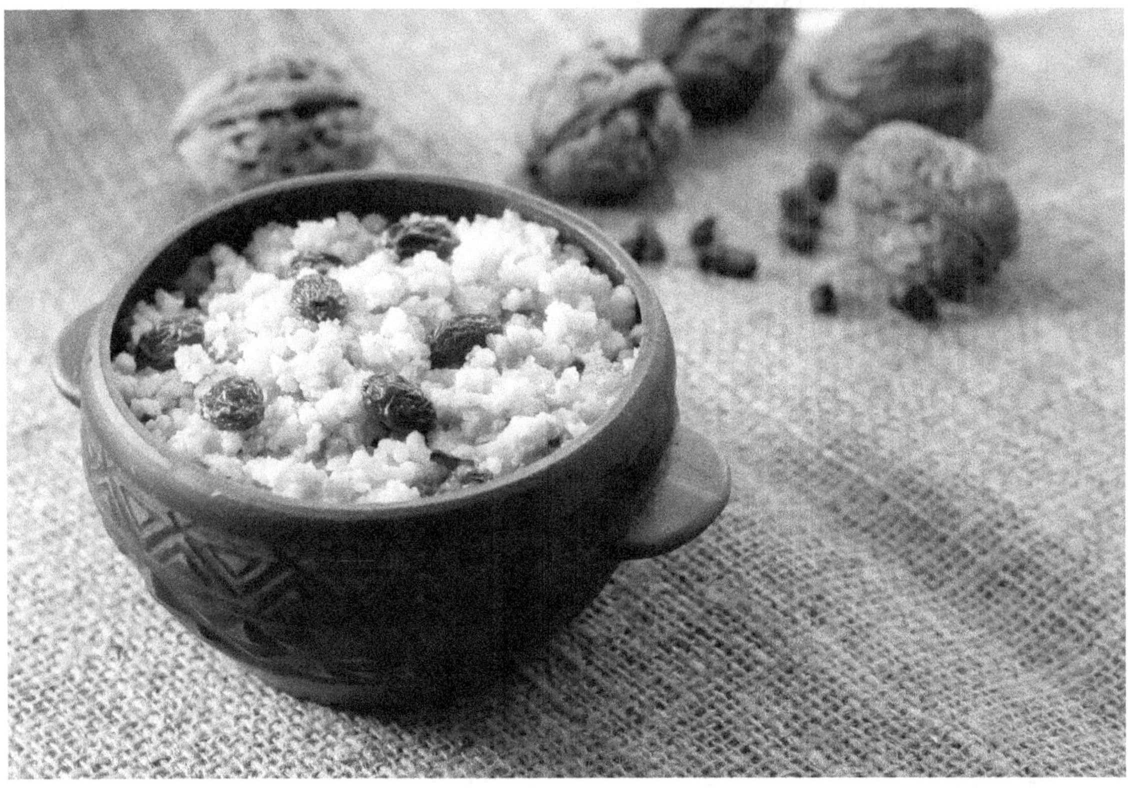

Millet Porridge is a wonderful porridge made from millet grits. Millet is a gluten-free nutritional powerhouse that is easy to prepare and is a great way to start your day.

Cook Time: 20 minutes

Servings: 2

Ingredients:

- Pinch of sea salt
- 1 tbsp. almonds, finely chopped
- ½ c. unsweetened almond milk
- ½ c. millet, rinsed and drained
- 1½ c. alkaline water
- 3 drops liquid stevia

Directions

Sauté millet in a non-stick skillet for 3 minutes.

Stir in salt and water. Let it boil, then reduce the heat.

Cook for 15 minutes, then stirs in remaining ingredients.

Cook for another 4 minutes.

Serve with chopped nuts on top.

Tofu Vegetable Fry

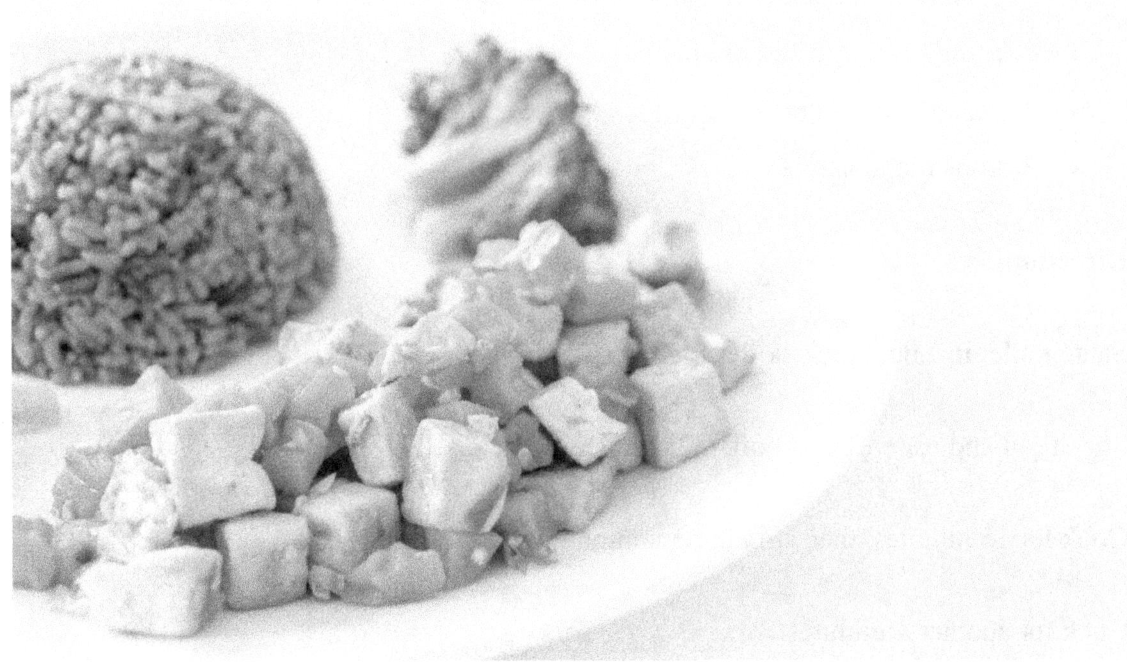

Tofu Vegetable Fry is a healthy alternative to conventional eating. This tasty recipe is vegan and easy to make.

Cook Time: 25 minutes

Servings: 4

Ingredients:

- 2 small onions, finely chopped
- 2 c. cherry tomatoes, finely chopped
- 1/8 tsp. ground turmeric
- 1 tbsp. olive oil
- 2 red bell peppers, seeded and chopped
- 3 c. firm tofu, crumbled and chopped
- 1/8 tsp. cayenne pepper
- 2 tbsp. fresh basil leaves, chopped
- Salt, to taste

Directions

Sauté onions and bell peppers in a greased skillet for 5 minutes.

Stir in tomatoes and cook for 2 minutes.

Add turmeric, salt, cayenne pepper, and tofu.

Cook for 8 minutes.

Garnish with basil leaves.

Serve warm.

Spiced Quinoa Porridge

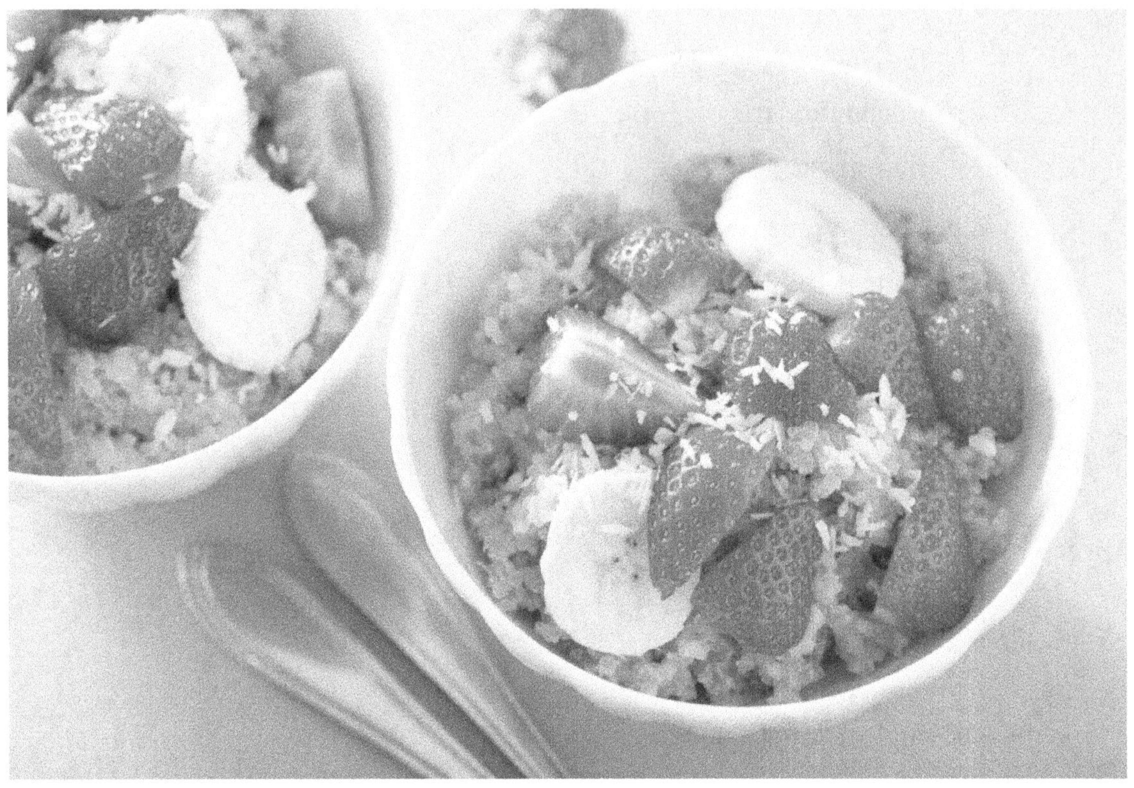

Spiced Quinoa Porridge is a very nutritious dish. The quinoa porridge recipe offers a great balance of flavors.

Cook time: 25 minutes

Servings: 4

Ingredients:

- 1 c. uncooked red quinoa, rinsed and drained
- 2 c. water
- ½ tsp. organic vanilla extract
- ½ c. coconut milk
- ¼ tsp. fresh lemon peel, grated finely
- 12 drops liquid stevia
- 1 tsp. ground cinnamon
- ½ tsp. ground ginger
- ½ tsp. ground nutmeg
- Pinch of ground cloves
- 2 tbsp. almonds, chopped

Directions

In a large pan, mix together the quinoa, water, and vanilla extract over medium heat and allow to a boil.

Reduce the heat to low and simmer, covered for about 15 minutes or until there is the absorption of all liquid, stirring occasionally.

In the pan with the quinoa, add the coconut milk, lemon peel, stevia, and spices and stir to combine.

Immediately remove from the heat and use a fork to fluff your quinoa.

Divide the quinoa mixture evenly into serving bowls.

Serve with a topping of chopped almonds.

Buckwheat Porridge

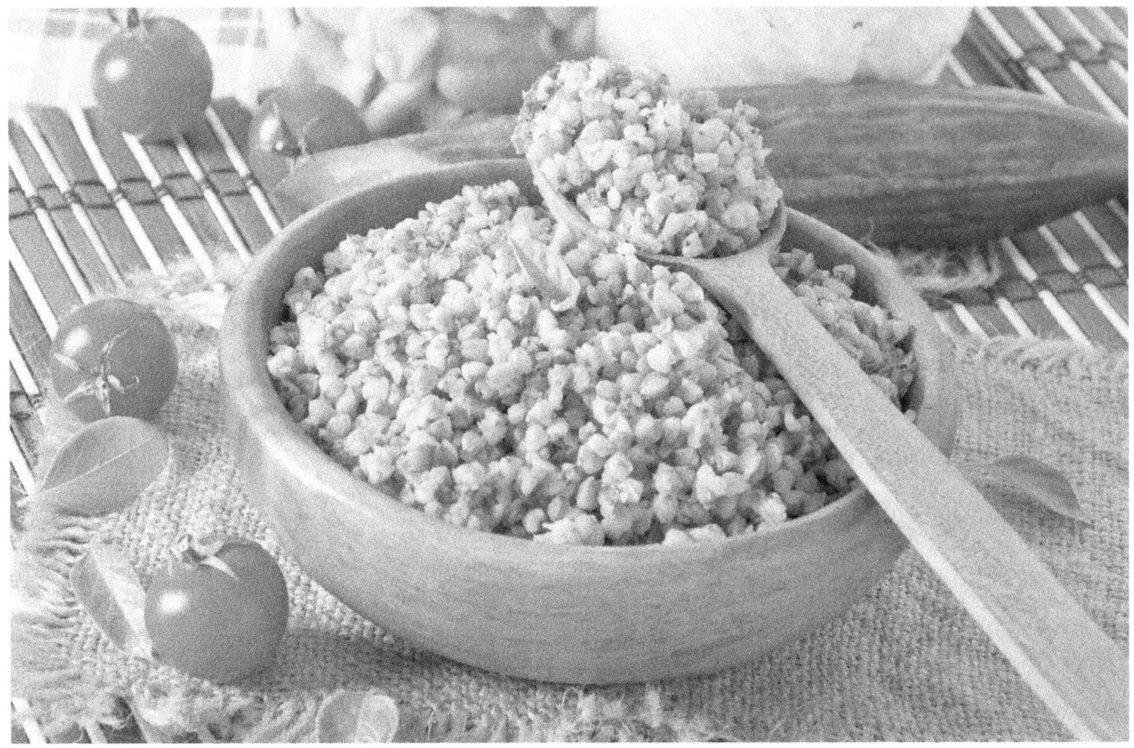

Buckwheat Porridge is a delicious gluten-free savory breakfast that is very easy to prepare. Made from buckwheat, it is a great addition to your superfood pantry.

Cook time: 15 minutes

Servings: 2

Ingredients:

- ½ c. buckwheat groats
- 2 tbsp. chia seeds
- 20 almonds
- 1 c. unsweetened almond milk
- ½ tsp. ground cinnamon
- 1 tsp. organic vanilla extract
- 4 drops liquid stevia
- ¼ c. mixed fresh berries

Directions

In a large bowl, soak buckwheat groats in 1 cup of water overnight.

In another 2 bowls, soak chia seeds and almonds respectively.

Drain the buckwheat and rinse well.

In a non-stick pan, add the buckwheat and almond milk over medium heat and cook for about 7 minutes or until creamy.

Drain the chia sees and almonds well.

Remove the pan from heat and stir in the almonds, chia seeds, cinnamon, vanilla extract, and stevia.

Serve hot with a topping of berries.

Overnight Fruity Oatmeal

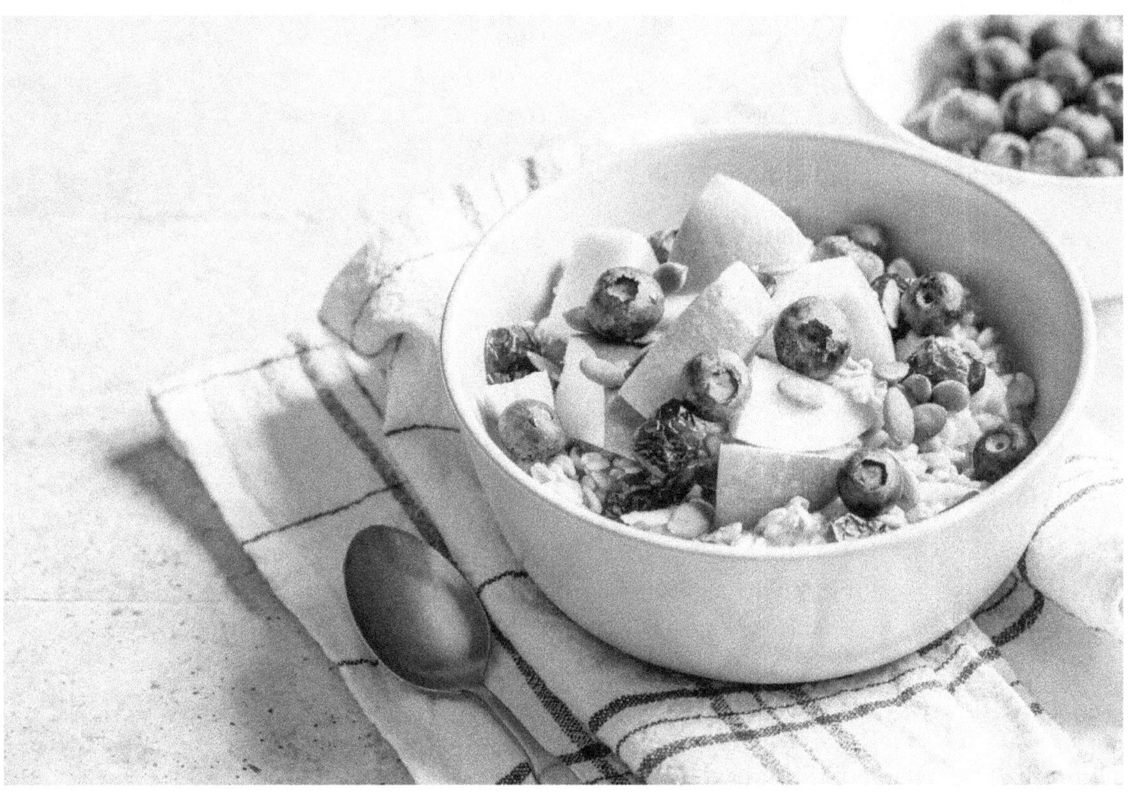

Overnight Fruity Oatmeal is a vegan, delicious, quick and easy breakfast that is great for kids. It combines gluten-free rolled oats, chopped fruit, and a delicious natural sweetener.

Cook time: 10 minutes

Servings: 2

Ingredients:

- 1 c. rolled oats
- 1 large banana, peeled and mashed
- 3 tsp. chia seeds
- 1 c. unsweetened almond milk
- ¼ c. fresh blueberries
- 2 tbsp. walnuts, chopped

Directions

In a large bowl, add all the ingredients except for sliced blueberries and walnuts and mix well until combined.

Cover the bowl and refrigerate overnight.

Top with blueberries and walnuts and serve.

Banana Waffles

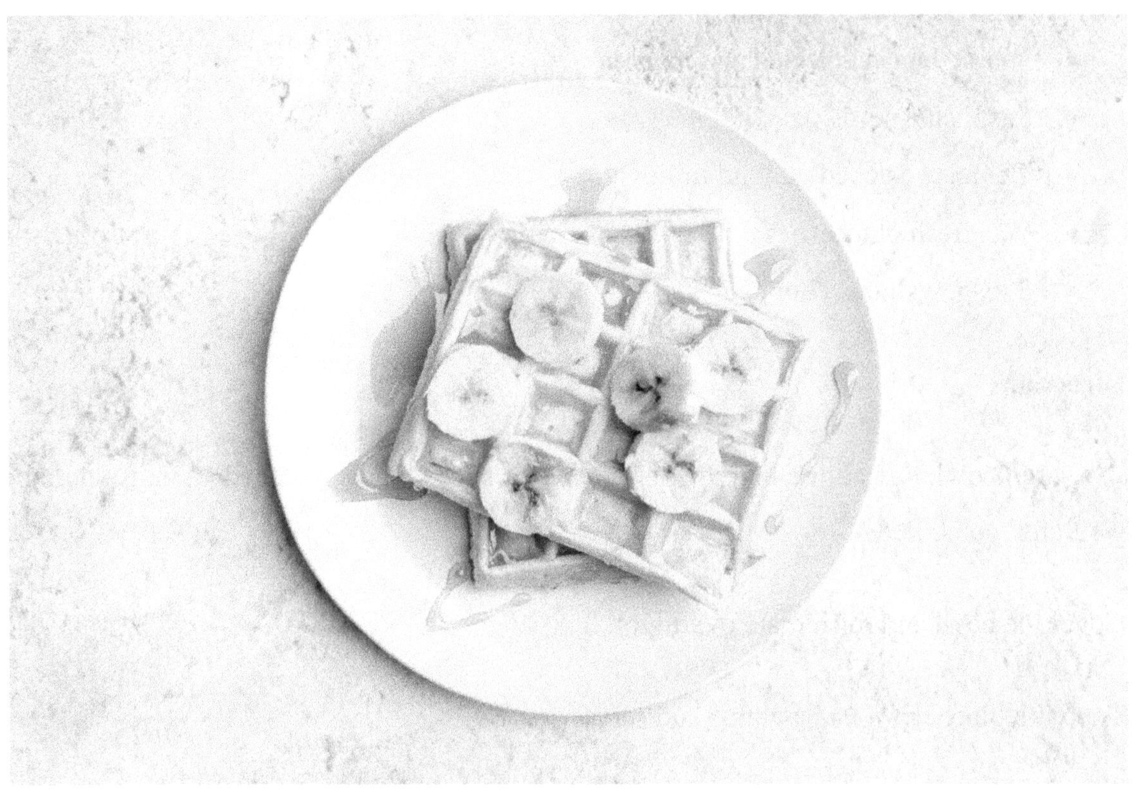

Banana Waffles are one of the most popular gluten-free, vegan waffle recipes on the Internet. Made from flax meal, bananas, and coconut milk among other ingredients, this recipe is as easy as 1-2-3.

Cook time: 35 minutes

Servings: 5

Ingredients:

- 2 tbsp. flax meal
- 6 tbsp. warm water
- 2 bananas, peeled and mashed
- 1 c. creamy almond butter
- ¼ c. full-fat coconut milk

Directions

In a small bowl, add the flax meal and warm water and beat until well combined.

Set aside for about 10 minutes or until mixture becomes thick.

In a medium mixing bowl, add the bananas, almond butter, and coconut milk, mix well.

Add the flax meal mixture and mix until well combined.

Preheat the waffle iron and lightly grease it.

Place the desired amount of the mixture in the preheated waffle iron.

Cook for about 3-4 minutes or until waffles become golden brown.

Repeat with the remaining mixture.

Serve warm.

Buckwheat Pancakes

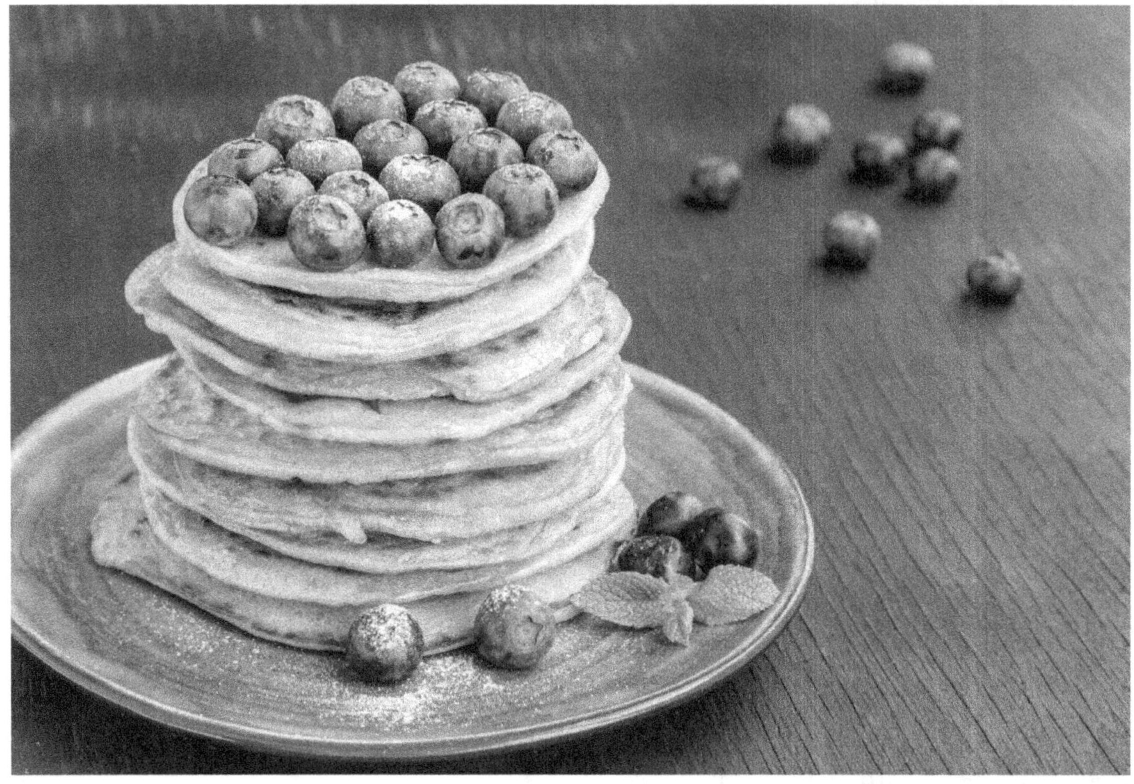

Buckwheat Pancakes are served with pear syrup. This is a delicious pole and open-faced savory pancake recipe. It seals in the flavors and is perfect for serving on Shabbat mornings.

Cook time: 15 minutes

Servings: 5

Ingredients:

- 1 c. coconut milk
- 1 tbsp. baking powder
- 2 tsp. apple cider vinegar
- ¼ tsp. sea salt
- 1 c. buckwheat flour
- 2 tbsp. ground flax seed
- ¼ c. maple syrup
- 1 tsp. vanilla extract
- 1 tbsp. coconut oil

Directions

In a medium bowl, mix the coconut milk and vinegar. Set aside.

In a separate bowl, mix together the flour, salt, flax seed, and baking powder.

Add the coconut milk mixture, vanilla, maple syrup, and beat well to combine.

In a large non-stick skillet, melt the coconut oil over medium high heat.

Place about ⅓ cup of the mixture and spread in an even circle.

Cook for about 1-2 minutes.

Flip and cook for an additional 1 minute then remove from pan.

Repeat with the rest of the mixture.

Serve warm.

Tomato Omelette

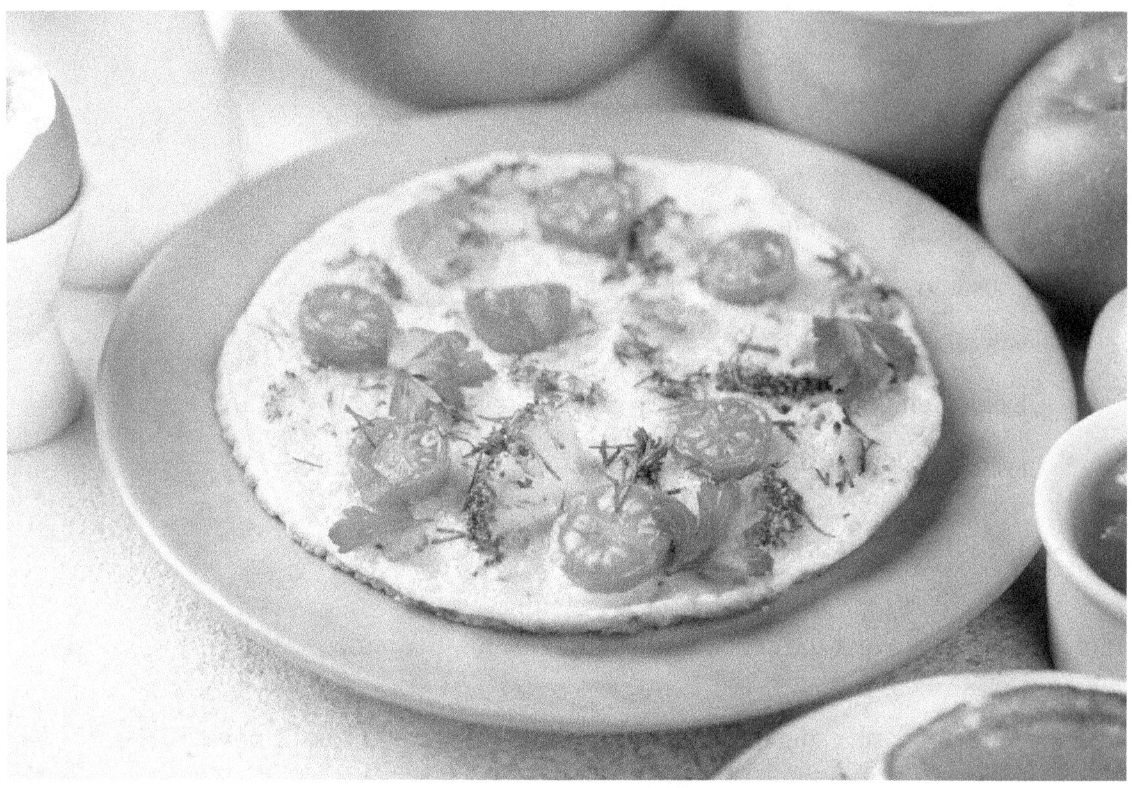

Tomato Omelette is a dish that is so easy to make. It is also easy to put in your toaster oven or a slow cooker. Let's try it!

Cook time: 25 minutes

Servings: 4

Ingredients:

- 1 c. chickpea flour
- ¼ tsp. ground turmeric
- ¼ tsp. red chili powder
- Pinch of ground cumin
- Pinch of salt
- 2 c. water
- 1 medium onion, chopped finely
- 2 medium tomatoes, chopped finely
- 1 jalapeño pepper, chopped finely
- 2 tbsp. fresh cilantro, chopped
- 2 tbsp. olive oil, divided

Directions

In a large bowl, mix together the flour, spices, and salt.

Slowly add the water and mix until well combined.

Add the onion, tomatoes, green chili, and cilantro and gently stir to combine.

In a large non-stick frying pan, heat ½ tbsp. of oil over medium heat.

Add ½ of tomato mixture and tilt the pan to spread it.

Cook for 5-7 minutes.

Pour remaining oil over the omelette and carefully flip to the other side.

Cook for 4-5 minutes or until golden brown and remove from pan.

Repeat with the remaining mixture.

Coconut & Nut Granola

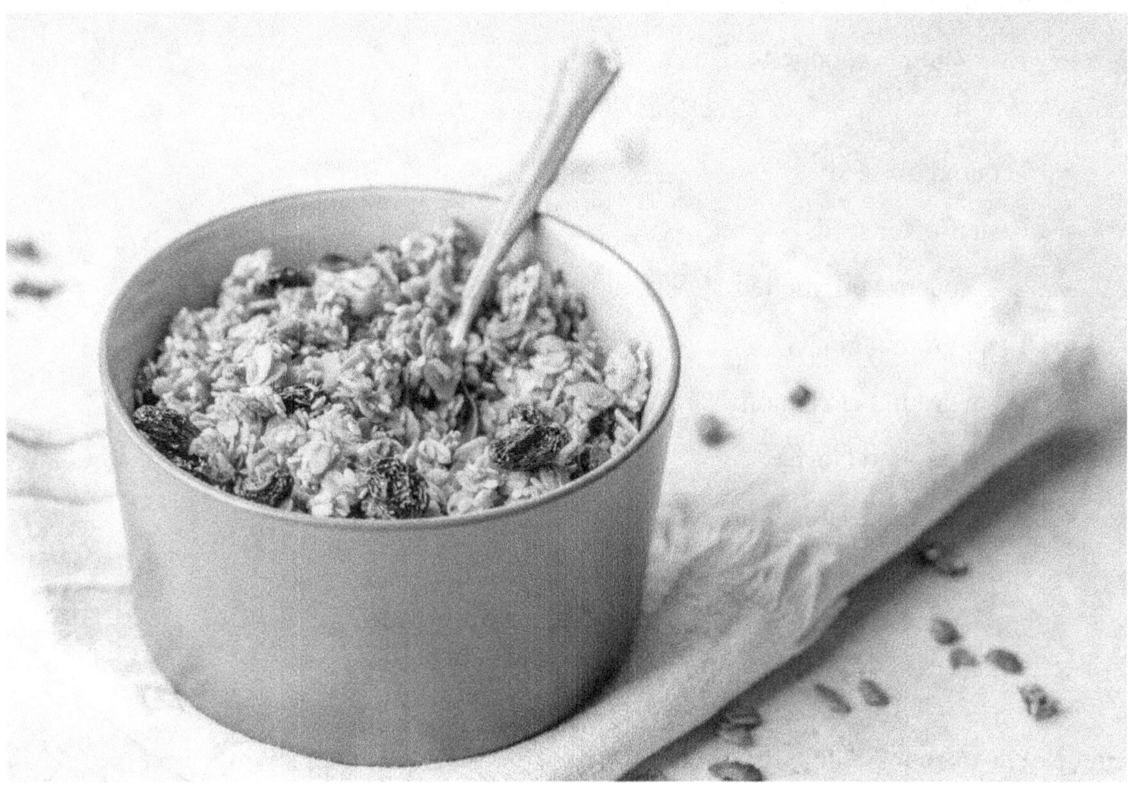

Coconut & Nut Granola is a savory granola recipe made from coconut, flaxseeds, sunflower, and pumpkin seeds. This recipe is dedicated to the holiday of Pesach because many of the ingredients are kosher for Passover.

Cook time: 30 minutes

Servings: 12

Ingredients:

- 3 c. unsweetened coconut flakes
- 1 c. walnuts, chopped
- ½ c. flaxseeds
- ⅔ pumpkin seeds
- ⅔ sunflower seeds
- ¼ c. coconut oil, melted
- 1 tsp. ground ginger
- 1 tsp. ground cinnamon
- ⅛ tsp. ground cloves
- ⅛ tsp. ground cardamom
- Pinch of salt

Directions

Preheat the oven to 350 degrees F. Lightly grease a large, rimmed baking sheet.

In a bowl, add the coconut flakes, walnuts, flaxseeds, pumpkin seeds, sunflower seeds, coconut oil, spices, and salt and toss to coat well.

Transfer the mixture onto the prepared baking sheet and spread in an even layer.

Bake for about 20 minutes, stirring after every 3-4 minutes.

Remove the baking sheet from the oven and let the granola cool completely before serving.

Break the granola into desired sized chunks and serve with your favorite non-dairy milk.

Lunch and Dinner Recipes

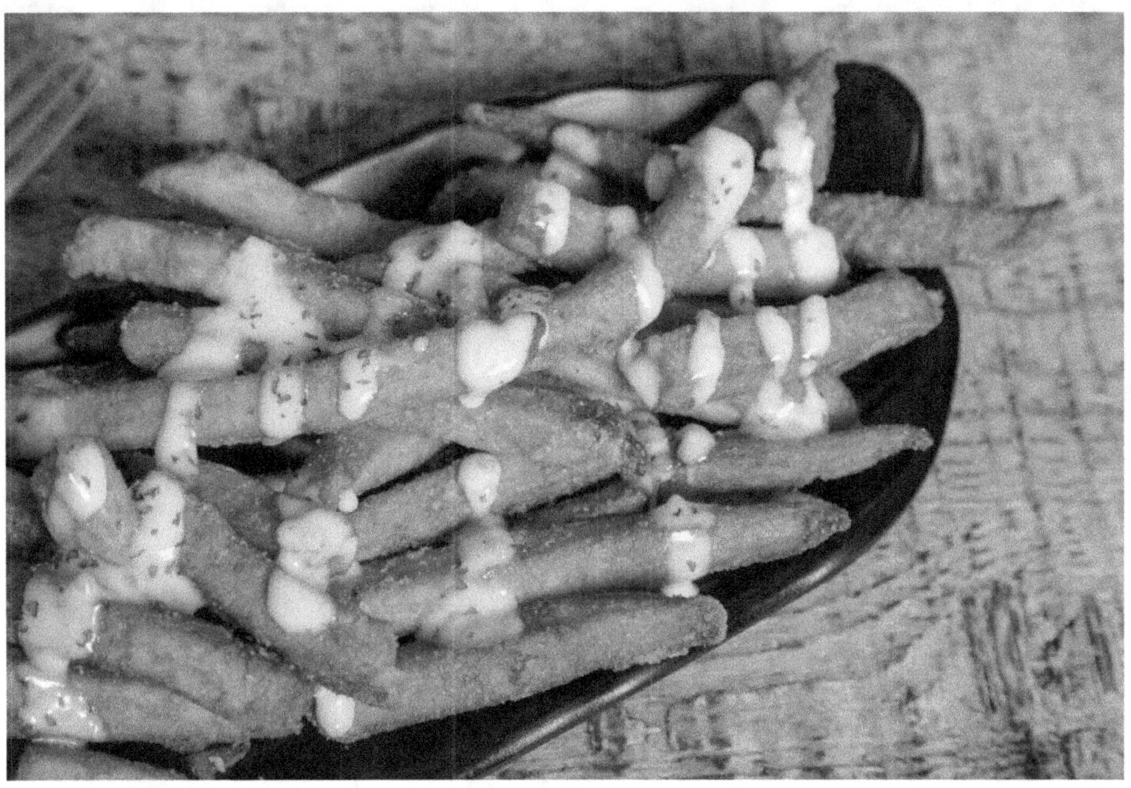

Lunch and Dinner Recipes are wonderful. They are easy to prepare, taste delicious, are affordable, and don't take long to make. The ingredients are easy to find and very affordable.

We all know that we have to eat more alkaline foods to achieve good health. But, often, we don't know how to incorporate them into our meals.

They are great recipes that are easy to make and taste delicious.

Enjoy!

Tomato & Greens Salad

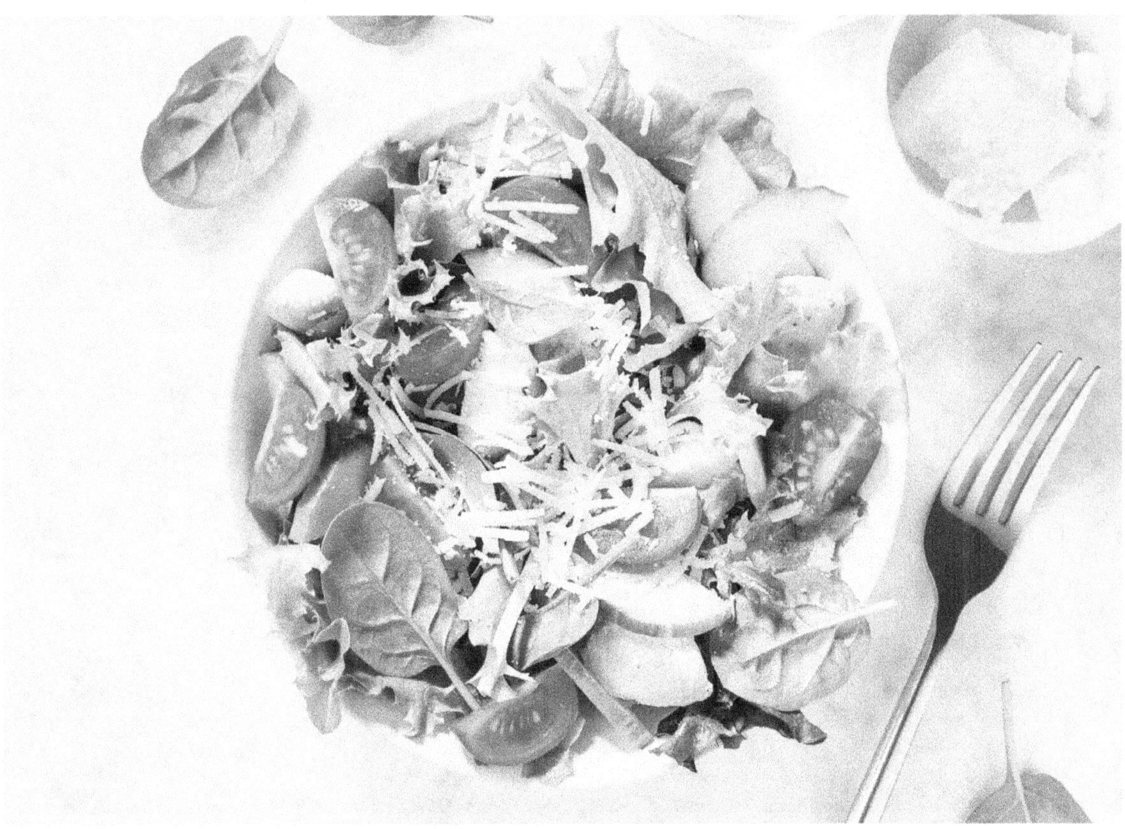

Tomato & Greens Salad is an awesome lunch or dinner salad. Just the right balance of veggie-acid-alkalies. You can substitute with canned tomatoes if it's too difficult to find fresh ones.

Cook time: 10 minutes

Servings: 4

Ingredients:

- 6 c. fresh baby greens
- 3 c. cherry tomatoes
- 2 tbsp. extra-virgin olive oil
- 1 tbsp. fresh lemon juice

Directions

In a large bowl, add all ingredients and toss to coat well.

Serve immediately.

Cucumber & Onion Salad

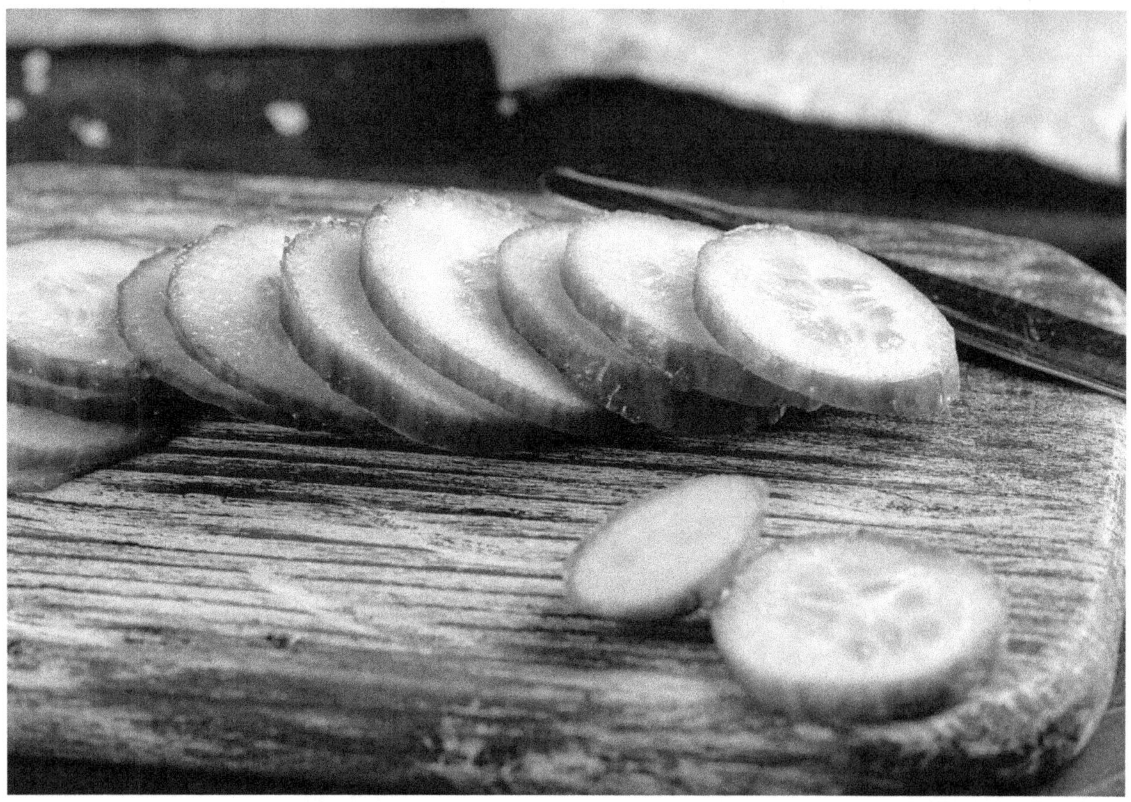

Cucumber & Onion Salad is an easy and delicious salad made with just a few ingredients. It's great for lunch or dinner. Don't forget to sprinkle with black pepper for the extra taste.

Cook time: 10 minutes

Servings: 5

Ingredients:

- 3 large cucumbers, sliced thinly
- ½ c. onion, sliced
- 2 tbsp. olive oil
- 1 tbsp. fresh apple cider vinegar
- Sea salt, to taste
- ¼ c. fresh cilantro, chopped

Directions

In a large bowl, add all ingredients and toss to coat well.

Serve immediately.

Apple Salad

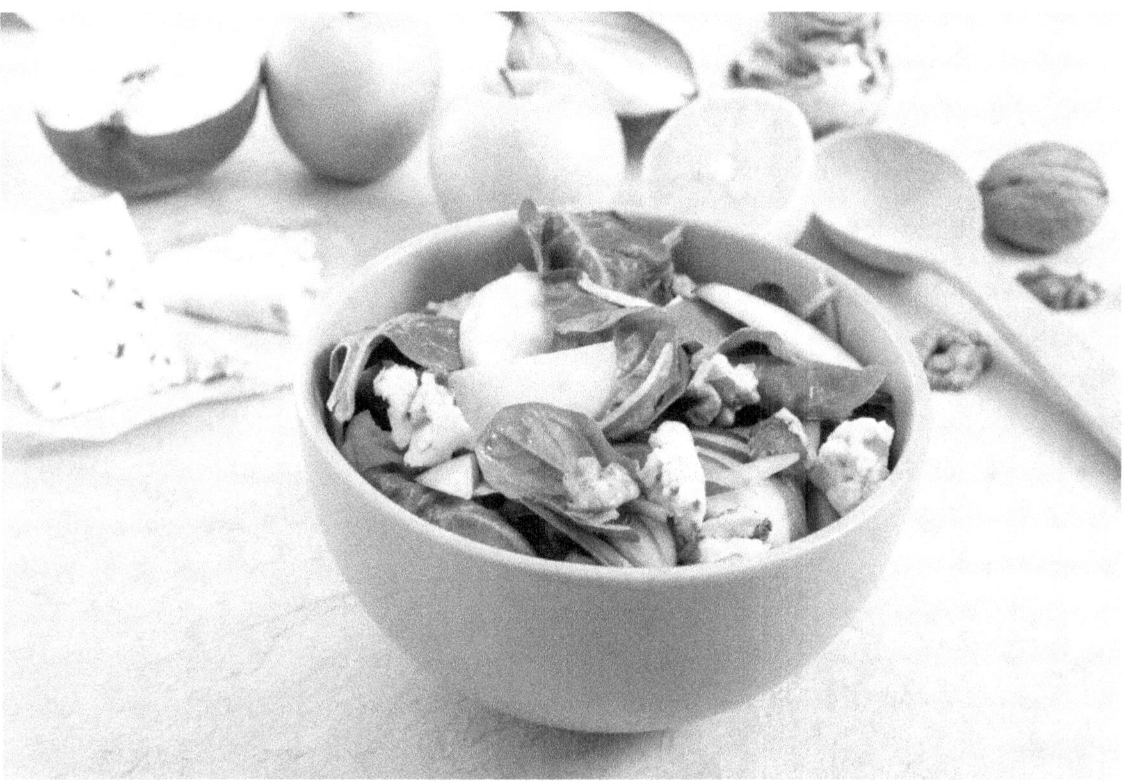

Apple Salad is a wonderful recipe. It's great as it provides a good amount of fiber. It's also a good source of calcium. It tastes good with any kind of marinade and with any kind of meat, or as a complete meal on its own. It can be used as a garnish for any dish.

Cook time: 10 minutes

Servings: 4

Ingredients:

- 4 large apples, cored and sliced
- 6 c. fresh baby spinach
- 3 tbsp. extra-virgin olive oil
- 2 tbsp. apple cider vinegar

Directions

In a large bowl, add all the ingredients and toss to coat well.

Serve immediately.

Okra Curry

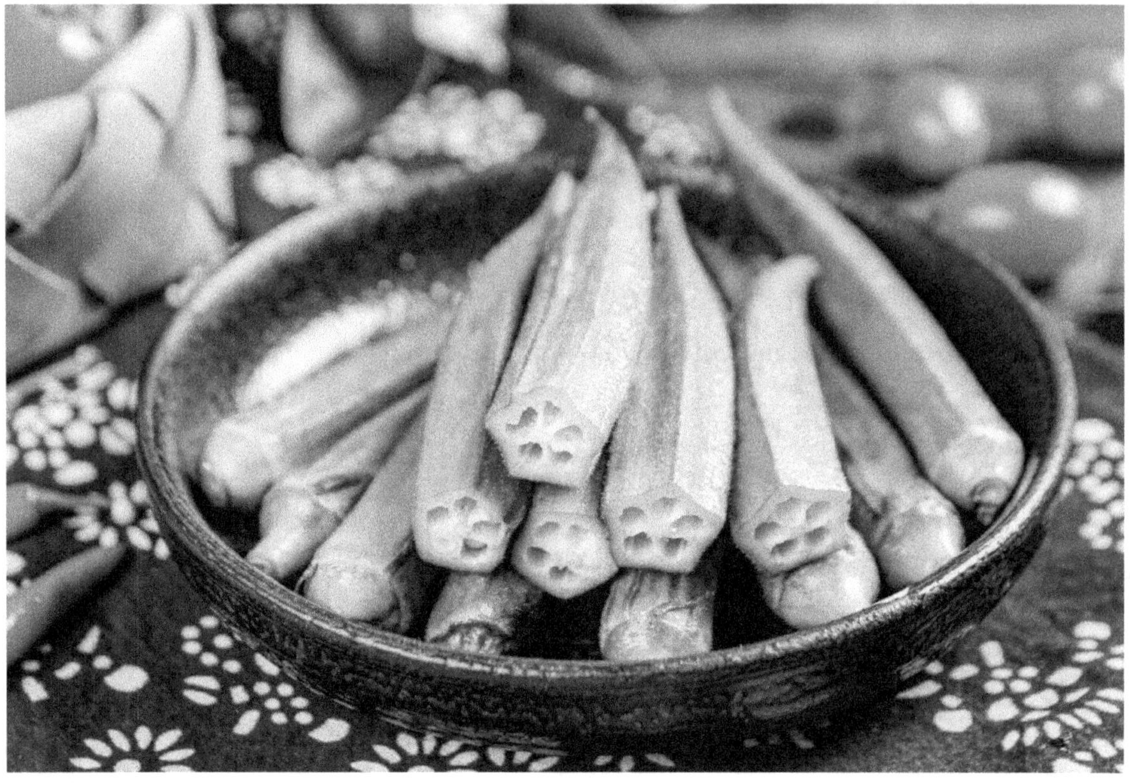

Okra Curry is delicious and a delightful curry great for any time of the day.

Cook time: 15 minutes

Servings: 2

Ingredients:

- 1 tbsp. olive oil
- ½ tsp. cumin seeds
- ½ tsp. red chili powder
- ¾ lb. trimmed okra pods, cut into 2-inch pieces
- 1 tsp. coriander, ground
- ½ tsp. curry powder
- Sea salt and freshly ground black pepper, to taste

Directions

In a skillet, add in oil and heat over medium heat and sauté the cumin seeds for 30 seconds.

Add the okra and stir fry for 1-1½ minutes.

Reduce the heat to low and cook, covered for 6-8 minutes, stirring occasionally.

Uncover and increase the heat to medium.

Stir in curry powder, red chili powder, and coriander and cook for 2-3 more minutes.

Season with salt and remove from heat.

Serve hot.

Vegetarian Burgers

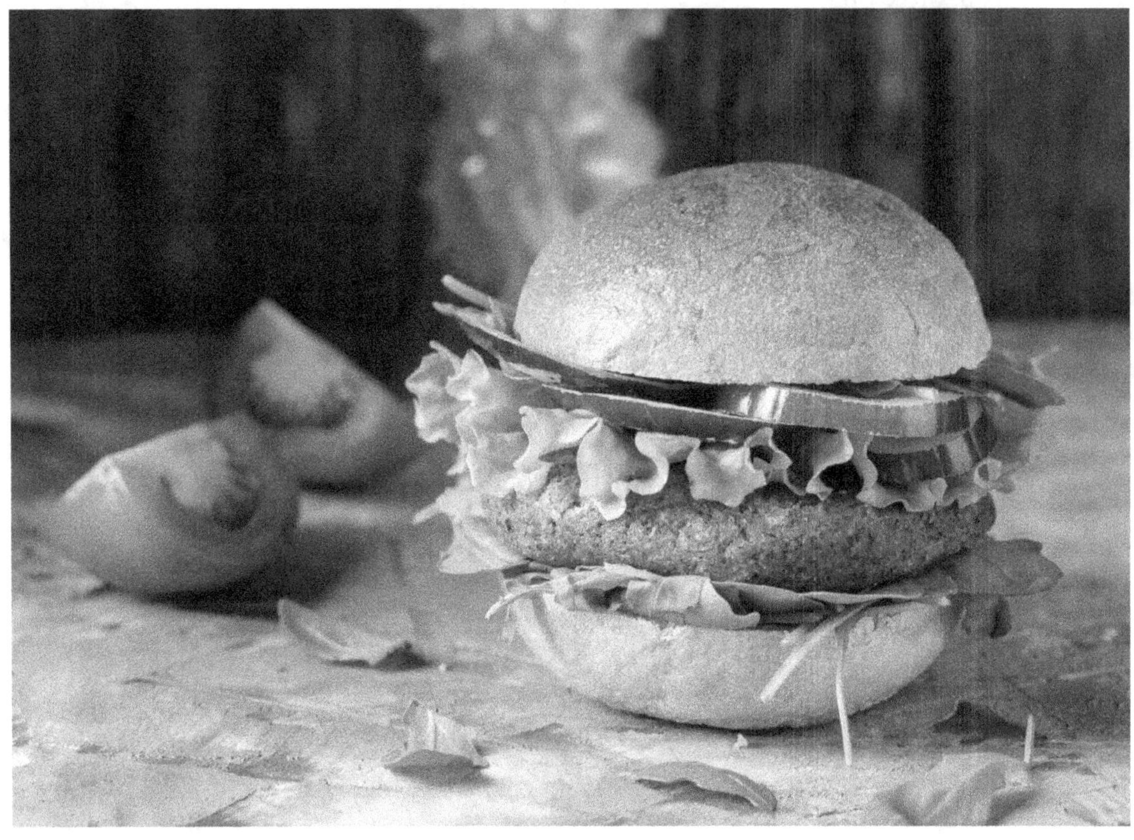

Vegetarian Burgers are healthy and tasty. They are a great alternative to traditional burgers and have a great variety of vegetable inclusion.

Cook time: 20 minutes

Servings: 4

Ingredients:

- 1 lb. firm tofu, drained, pressed, and crumbled
- ¾ c. rolled oats
- ¼ c. flaxseeds
- 2 c. frozen spinach, thawed
- 1 medium onion, chopped finely
- 4 garlic cloves, minced
- 1 tsp. ground cumin
- 1 tsp. red pepper flakes, crushed
- Sea salt and freshly ground black pepper, to taste
- 2 tbsp. olive oil
- 6 c. fresh salad greens

Directions

In a large bowl, add all the ingredients except oil and salad greens and mix until well combined.

Set aside for about 10 minutes.

Make desired size patties from mixture.

In a nonstick frying pan, heat the oil over medium heat and cook the patties for 6-8 minutes per side.

Serve these patties alongside the salad greens.

Eggplant Curry

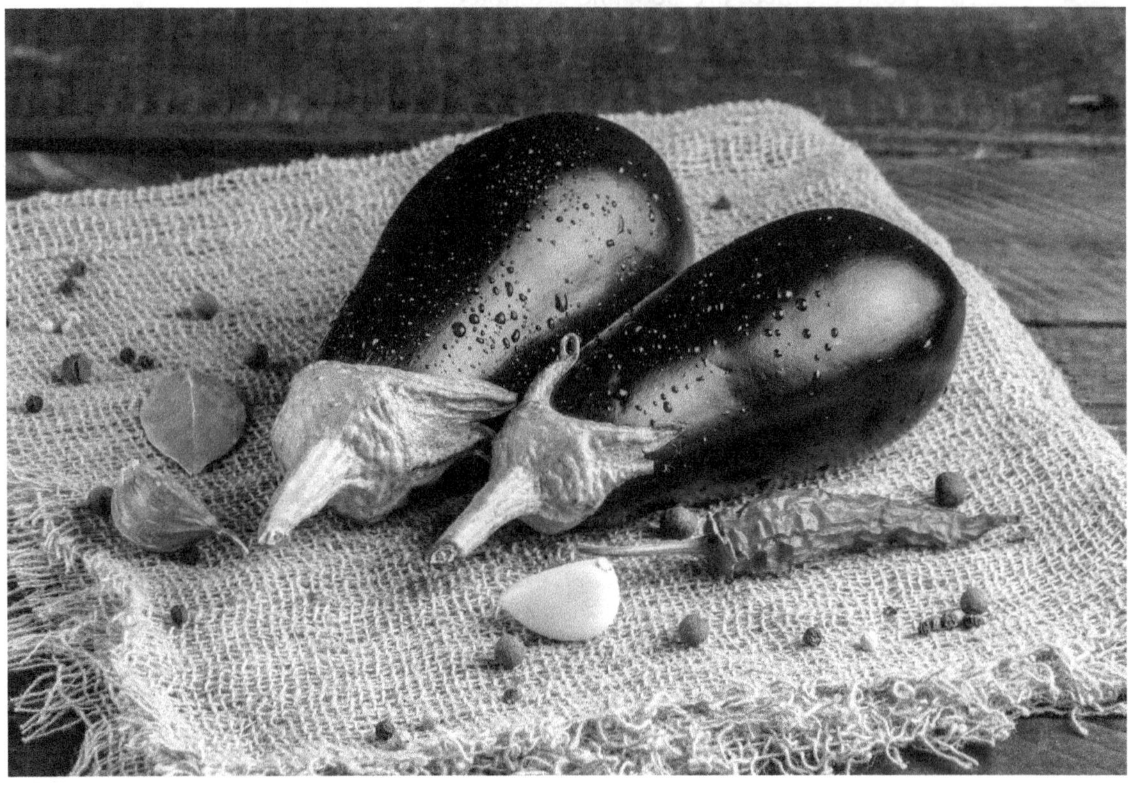

Eggplant Curry is one of the most flavorful curries there is. When you pair it with rice, it is a complete meal!

Cook time: 50 minutes

Servings: 3

Ingredients:

- 1 tbsp. coconut oil
- 1 medium onion, chopped finely
- 2 garlic cloves, minced
- ½ tbsp. fresh ginger, minced
- 1 Serrano pepper, seeded and minced
- 1 tsp. curry powder
- ¼ tsp. cayenne pepper
- Sea salt, to taste
- 1 medium tomato, finely chopped
- 1 large eggplant, cubed
- 1 c. unsweetened coconut milk
- 2 tbsp. fresh cilantro, chopped

Directions

In a large skillet, melt the coconut oil over medium heat and sauté the onion for 8-9 minutes.

Add the garlic, garlic, Serrano pepper, curry powder, cayenne pepper, and salt and sauté for 1 minute.

Add the tomato and cook for 3-4 minutes, crushing with the back of spoon.

Add the eggplant and salt and cook for 1 minute, stirring occasionally.

Stir in the coconut milk and bring to a gentle boil.

Reduce the heat to medium-low and simmer, covered for 15-20 minutes or until done completely.

Serve with a garnish of cilantro.

Rosemary Roasted Yams

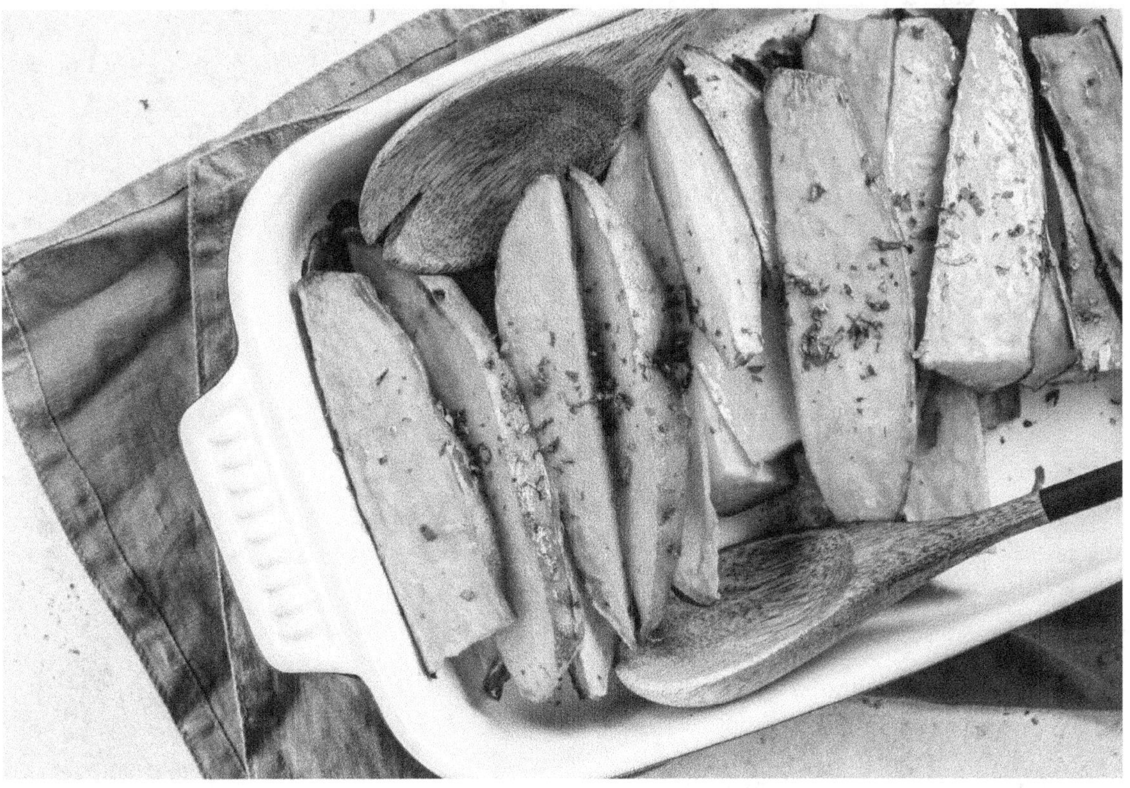

Rosemary Roasted Yams are a great healthy dish. The flavor of the yams is amazing and adds a whole new dimension when blended with fresh rosemary.

Cook time: 55 minutes

Servings: 4

Ingredients:

- 2 c. cubed yams
- 1 tbsp. coconut oil
- 6 fresh rosemary sprigs leave removed and finely chopped stems discarded
- Celtic sea salt, iodine-free, to taste
- Black pepper to taste

Directions

Preheat your oven to 375 degrees F.

Mix yams with rosemary and oil in a bowl.

Spread the yams on a baking sheet.

Bake for 45 to 50 minutes.

Adjust seasoning with salt and pepper.

Serve warm.

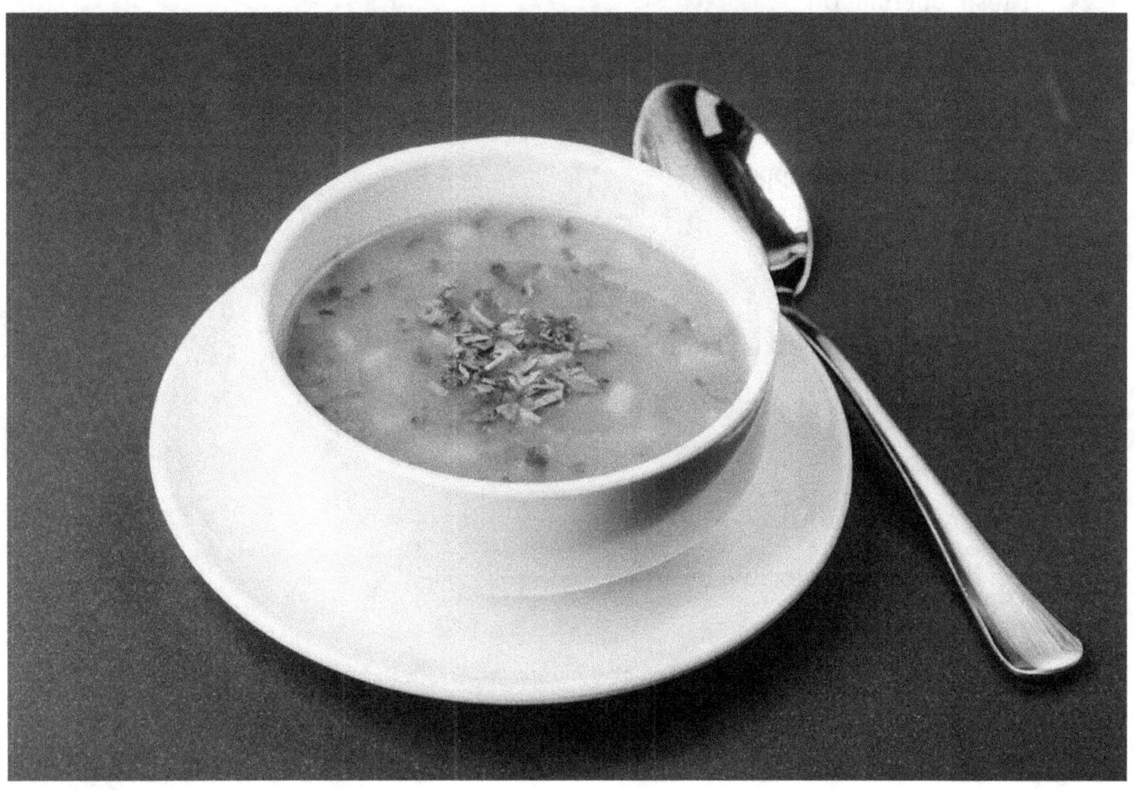

Quinoa & Lentil Soup is a hearty soup that is packed full of nutrients, making it a great meal to have throughout the day.

Cook time: 40 minutes

Servings: 6

Ingredients:

- 1 tbsp. coconut oil
- 3 carrots, peeled and chopped
- 3 celery stalks, chopped
- 1 yellow onion, chopped
- 4 garlic cloves, minced
- 4 c. tomatoes, chopped
- 1 c. red lentils, rinsed and drained
- ½ c. dried quinoa, rinsed and drained
- 1½ tsp. ground cumin
- 1 tsp. red chili powder
- 6 c. homemade vegetable broth
- 2 c. fresh spinach, chopped

Directions

In a large pan, heat the oil over medium heat and sauté the celery, onion, and carrot for 4-5 minutes.

Add the garlic and sauté for about 1 minute.

Add the remaining ingredients except spinach and bring to a boil.

Reduce the heat to low and simmer, covered for 20 minutes.

Stir in spinach and simmer for 3-4 minutes.

Serve hot.

Lentil & Veggie Soup

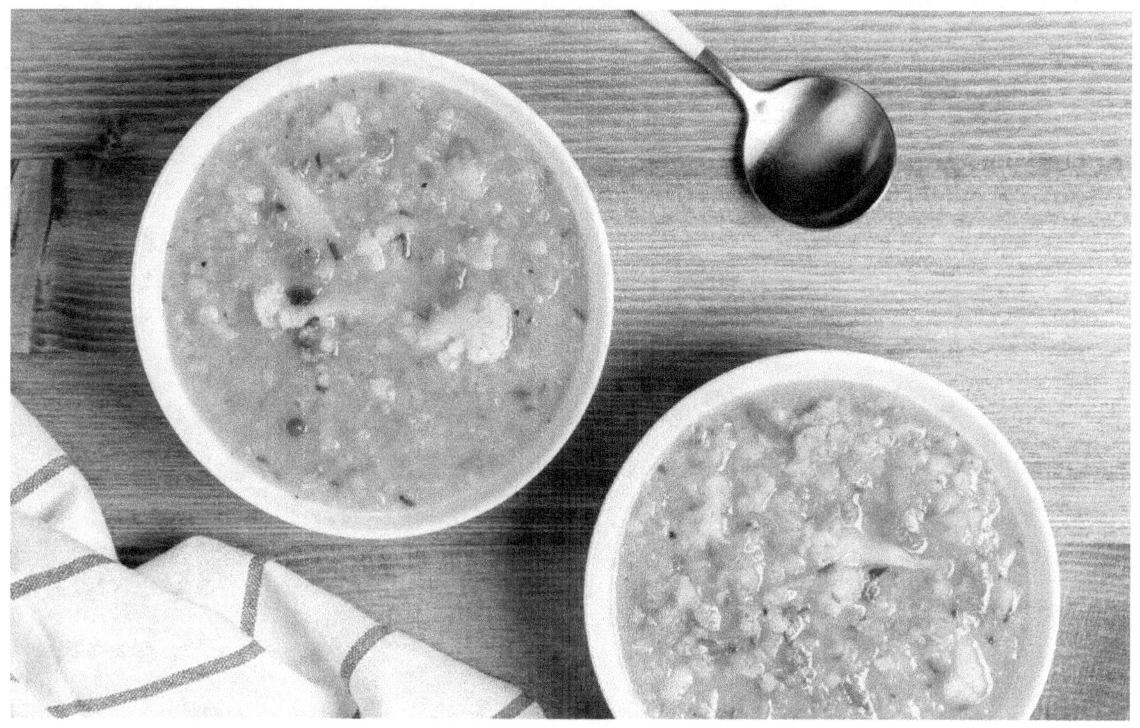

Lentil & Veggie Soup is another wonderful soup. It's very hearty and healthy.

Cook time: 1 hour 30 minutes

Servings: 8

Ingredients:

- 2 tbsp. olive oil
- 2 carrots, peeled and chopped
- 2 celery stalks, chopped
- 2 sweet onions, chopped
- 3 garlic cloves, minced
- 1¾ c. brown lentils, rinsed
- 2½ c. tomatoes, finely chopped
- ¼ tsp. dried basil, crushed
- ¼ tsp. crushed oregano, dried
- ¼ tsp. crushed thyme, dried
- 1 tsp. ground cumin
- ½ tsp. ground coriander
- ½ tsp. paprika
- 6 c. homemade vegetable broth
- 3 c. fresh spinach, chopped
- Sea salt and freshly ground black pepper
- 2 tbsp. fresh lemon juice

Directions

In a soup pan, add the oil and heat over medium heat and sauté carrot, celery, and onion for 5 minutes.

Add the garlic, sauté for about 1 minute.

Add the lentils and sauté for 3 minutes.

Stir in the tomatoes, herbs, spices, and broth and allow to a boil.

Reduce the heat to low and simmer, partially covered for about 1 hour or until desired doneness

Stir in the spinach, salt and black pepper and cook for 4 minutes.

Stir in the lemon juice and serve hot.

Mixed Mushroom Stew

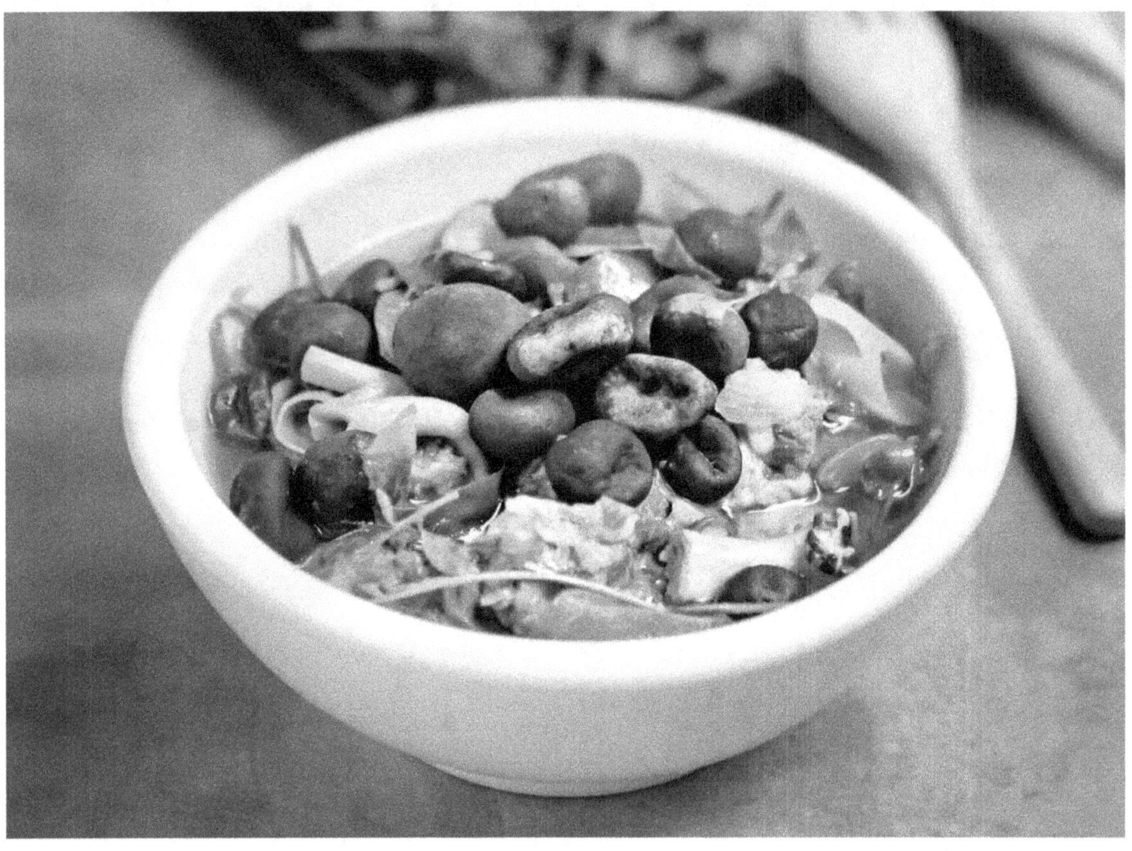

Mixed Mushroom Stew is amazing! This stew is sure to have you coming back for more.

Cook time: 30 minutes

Servings: 4

Ingredients:

- 2 tbsp. olive oil
- 3 garlic cloves, minced
- 2 onions, chopped
- ½ lb. fresh button mushrooms, chopped
- ¼ lb. fresh shiitake mushrooms, chopped
- ¼ lb. fresh Portobello mushrooms, chopped
- Sea salt and freshly ground black pepper, to taste
- ¼ c. homemade vegetable broth
- ½ c. coconut milk
- 2 tbsp. fresh parsley, chopped

Directions

In a large skillet, heat oil over medium heat and sauté the onion and garlic for 4-5 minutes.

Add the mushrooms, salt, and black pepper and cook for 4-5 minutes.

Add the broth and coconut milk and bring to a gentle boil.

Simmer for 4-5 minutes or until desired doneness.

Stir in the cilantro and remove from heat.

Serve hot.

Lentil Chili

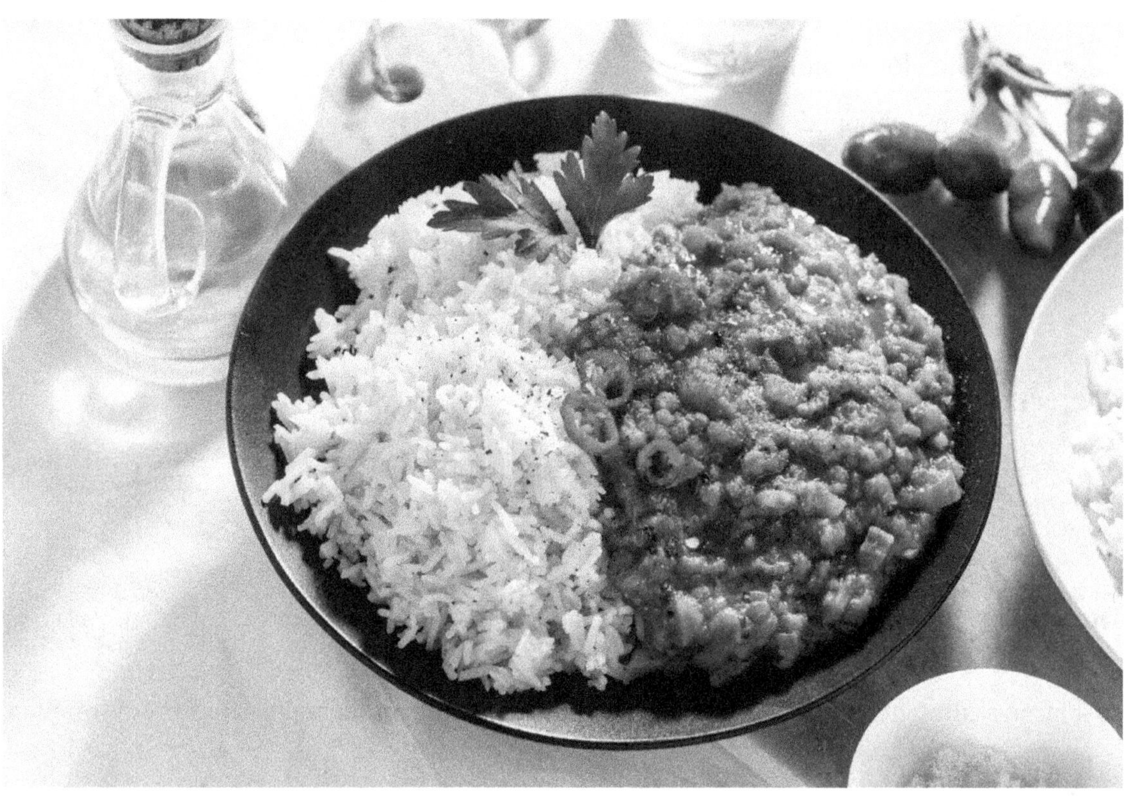

Lentil Chili is a good chili recipe that is also very healthy. It will be your new favorite for sure.

Cook time: 2 hours 55 minutes

Servings: 8

Ingredients:

- 2 tsp. olive oil
- 3 medium carrots, peeled and chopped
- 4 celery stalks, chopped
- 1 large onion, chopped
- 2 garlic cloves, minced
- 1 jalapeño pepper, seeded and chopped
- ½ tbsp. dried thyme, crushed
- 1 tbsp. chipotle chili powder
- ½ tbsp. cayenne pepper
- 1½ tbsp. ground coriander
- 1½ tbsp. ground cumin
- 1 tsp. ground turmeric
- Sea salt and freshly ground black pepper, to taste
- 1 lb. red lentils, rinsed
- 8 c. homemade vegetable broth
- ½ c. scallion, chopped

Directions

In a large pan, heat the oil over medium heat and sauté the onion, carrot, and celery for 5 minutes.

Add the garlic, jalapeño pepper, thyme, and spices and sauté for about 1 minute.

Add the tomato paste, lentils, and broth and bring to a boil.

Reduce the heat to low and simmer for 2-2½ hours.

Serve hot with a garnish of scallion.

Kidney Bean Curry

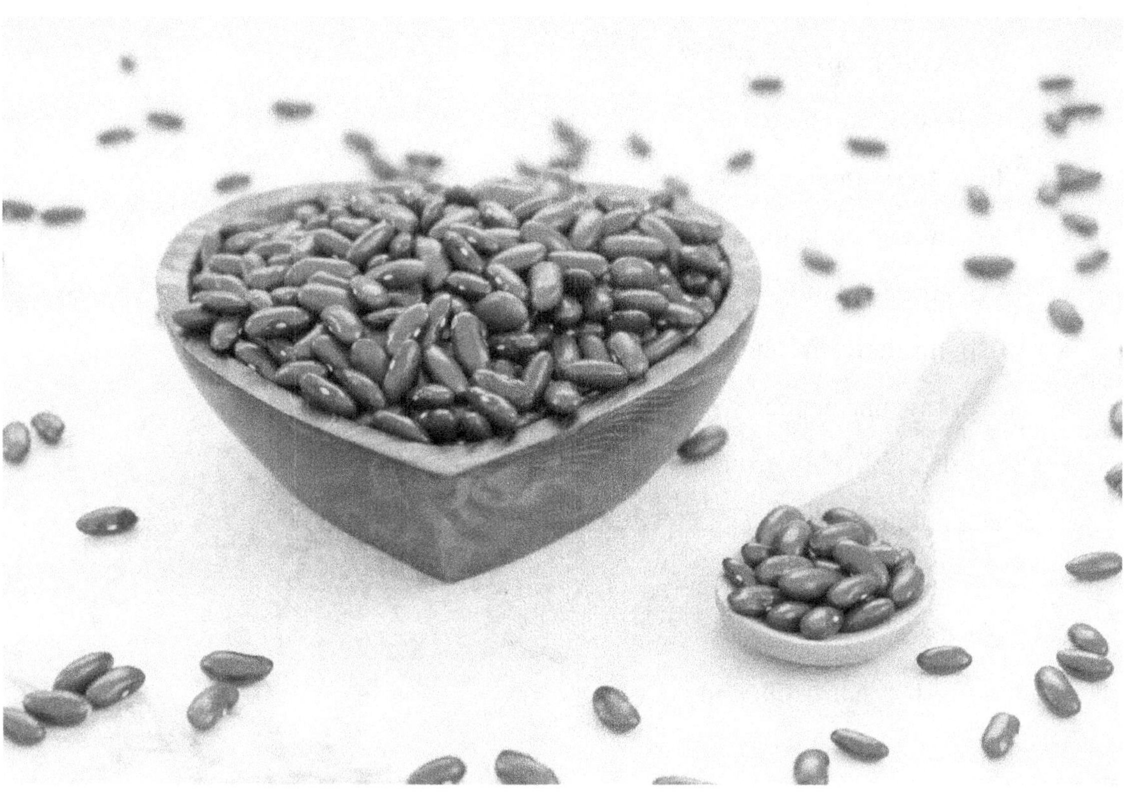

Kidney Bean Curry is wonderful world cuisine. It is made with just a few ingredients and the outcome is amazing. It's delicious when served with little white corn tortillas.

Cook time: 40 minutes

Servings: 6

Ingredients:

- 4 tbsps. olive oil
- 1 medium onion, chopped finely
- 2 garlic cloves, minced
- 2 tbsp. fresh ginger, minced
- 1 tsp. ground coriander
- 1 tsp. ground cumin
- ½ tsp. turmeric, ground
- ¼ tsp. cayenne pepper
- Sea salt and freshly ground black pepper, to taste
- 2 large plum tomatoes, chopped finely
- 3 c. cooked red kidney beans
- 2 c. water
- ¼ c. fresh cilantro, chopped

Directions

In a pan, add the oil and heat over medium high heat and allow the onion, garlic, and ginger to sauté for about 8 minutes.

Stir in the spices cook for about 1-2 minutes.

Stir in the tomatoes, kidney beans, and water and bring to a boil over high heat.

Decrease the heat to medium and simmer for 10-15 minutes or until desired thickness.

Serve hot with a garnish of parsley.

Smoothies

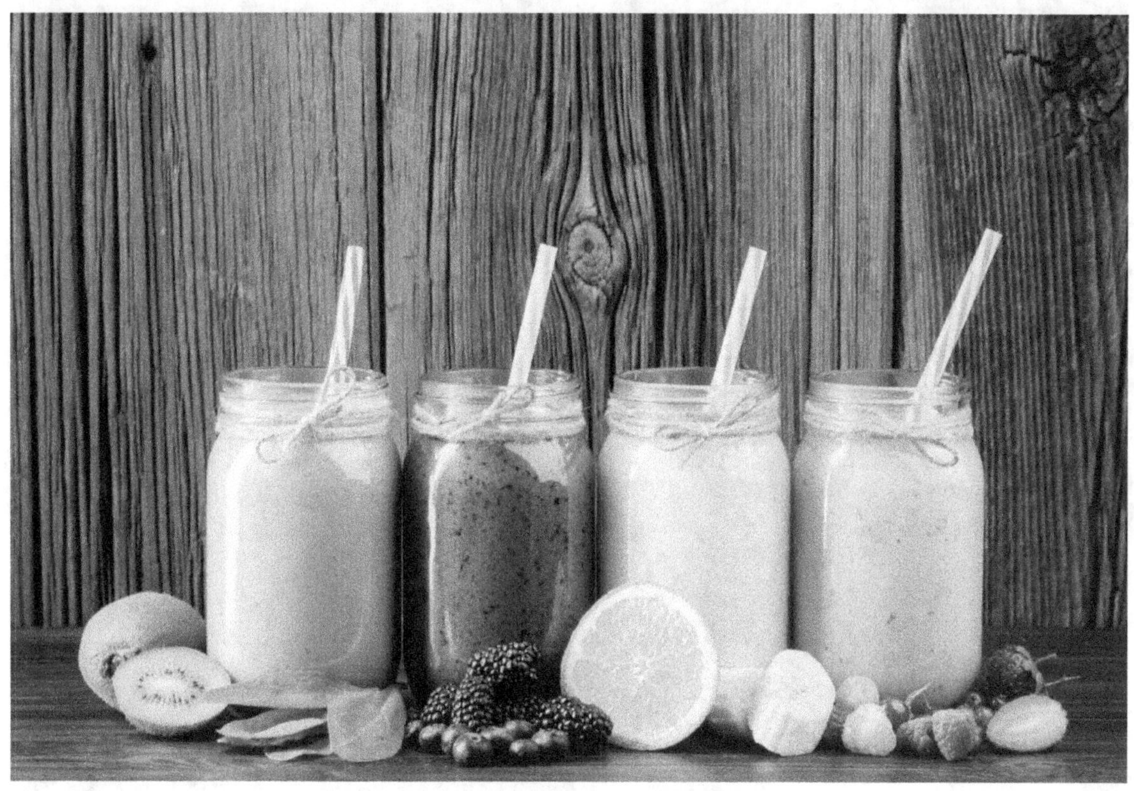

Smoothies. What are they exactly? Well, let's just say that they're not simply a beverage with a little bit of fiber in them...

Smoothies are the dietary key to attaining the beautiful "sunshine yellow" glow that you've always wanted. It's about the nutrients. It's about getting your daily intake of vegetables, fruits, and grains. Granola. Fruit. Protein. And all the good stuff that has been so elusive for so long.

Hearty Alkaline Strawberry Summer Deluxe

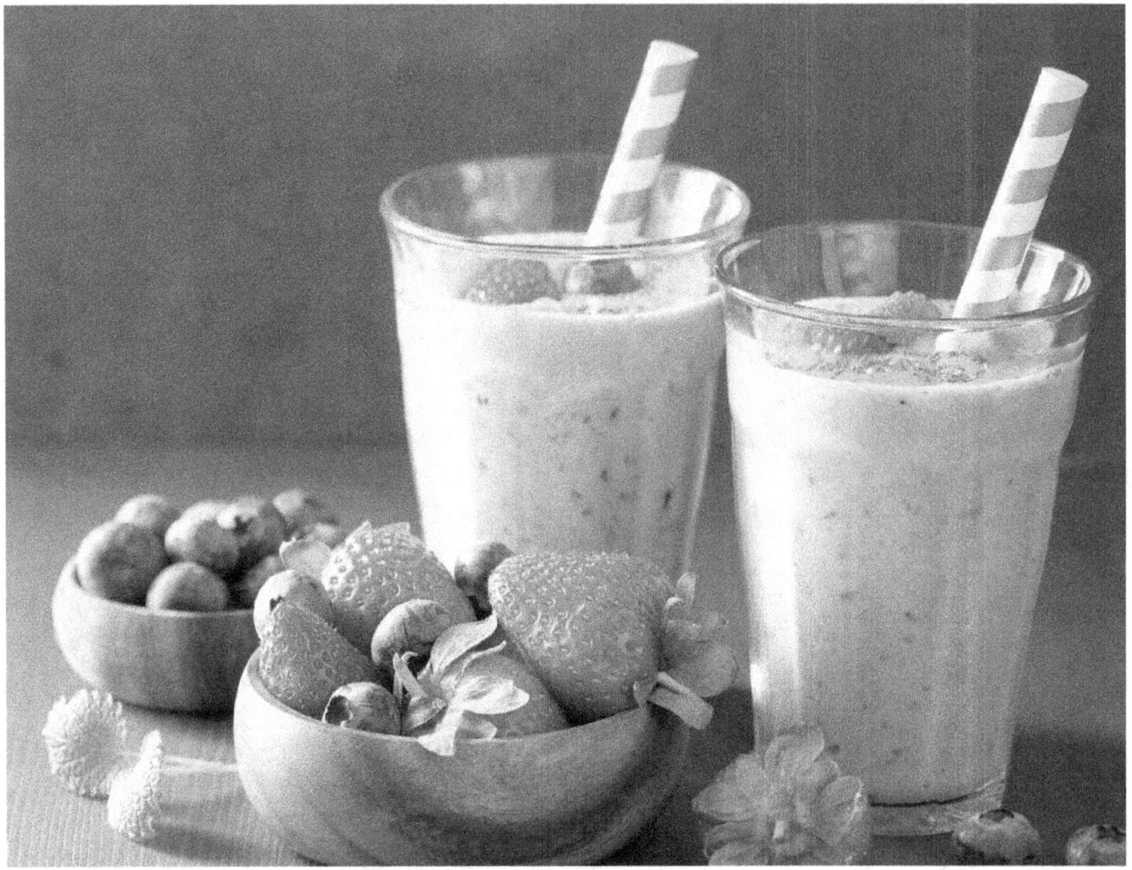

Hearty Alkaline Strawberry Summer Deluxe Smoothie is a nice way to start any summer morning. This smoothie is best made with fresh wild local strawberries, not with grocery store strawberries that have been shipped from far away from where they are not grown locally. Strawberries are in season during the summer and are most flavorful at that time.

Servings: 2

Cook Time: 5 minutes

Ingredients

- ½ c. organic strawberries/blueberries
- ½ banana
- 2 c. coconut water
- ½ inch ginger
- Juice of 2 grapefruits

Directions

Add all the listed ingredients to your blender

Blend until smooth

Add a few ice cubes and serve the smoothie

Enjoy!

Delish Pineapple and Coconut Milk Smoothie

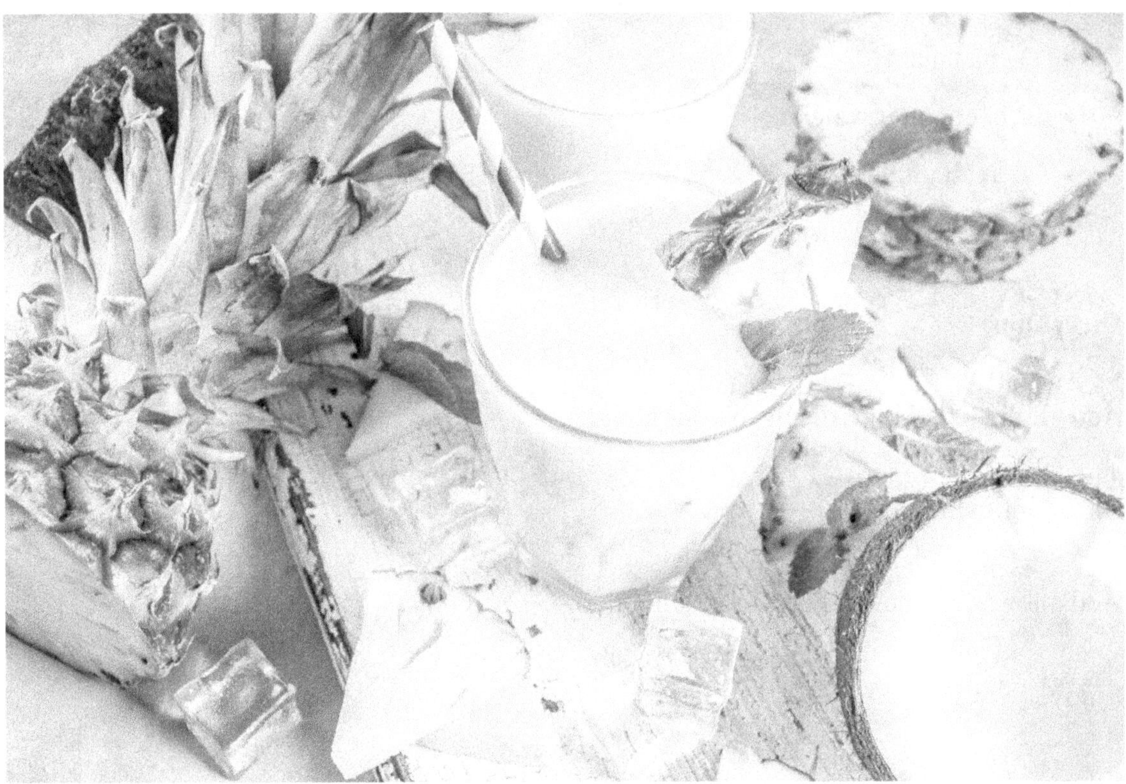

Delish Pineapple and Coconut Milk Smoothie is a great tropical smoothie for a summer afternoon treat. Pineapple contains powerful antioxidants, and coconut milk provides even more antioxidants. This is a delicious smoothie that is tasty any time of the year.

Servings: 2

Cook Time: 5 minutes

Ingredients

- ¼ c. frozen pineapple
- ¾ c. coconut milk

Directions

Add the listed ingredients to your blender and blend well with settings on high

Once the mixture is smooth, pour smoothie in a tall glass and serve

Chill and enjoy!

Cabbage and Coconut Chia Smoothie

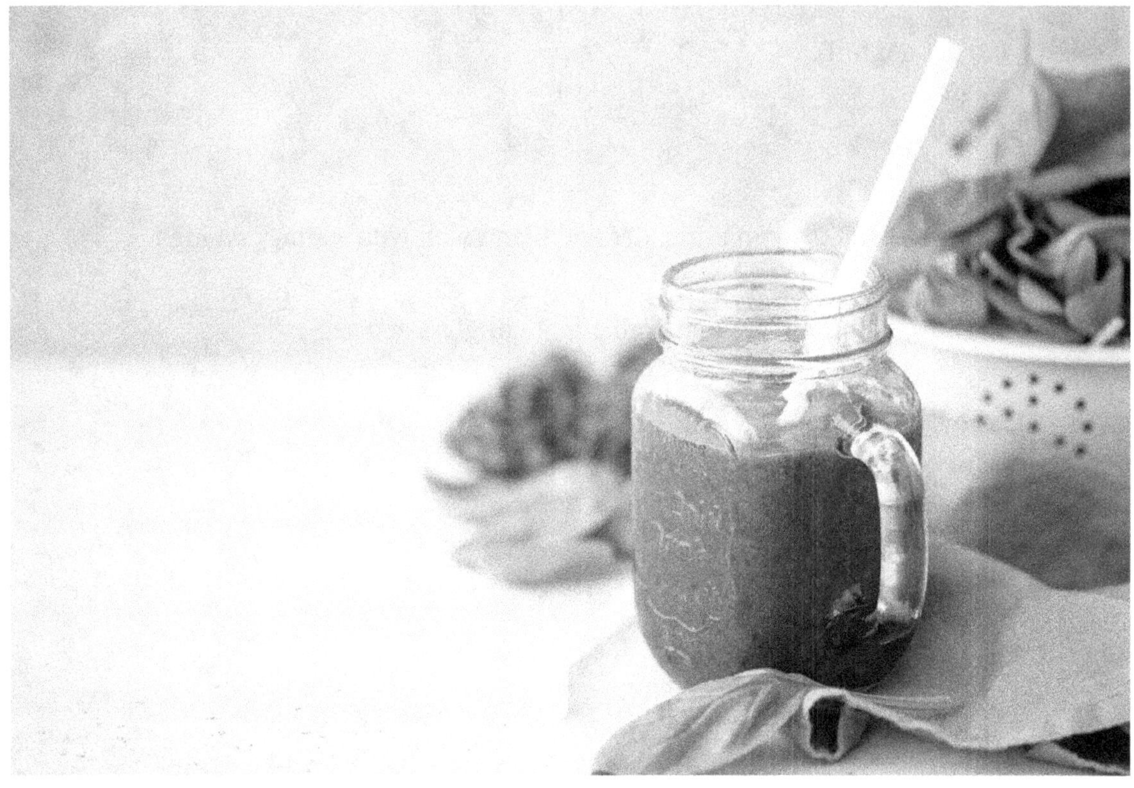

Cabbage and Coconut Chia Smoothie is a great alkaline smoothie loaded with antioxidants. It is a sweet treat with a healthy twist. It is a great way to add more greens to your diet because it tastes so good with the cherries.

Servings: 2

Cook Time: 5 minutes

Ingredients

- 1/3 c. cabbage
- 1 c. cold unsweetened coconut milk
- 1 tbsp. chia seeds
- ½ c. cherries
- ½ c. spinach

Directions

Add coconut milk to your blender

Cut cabbage and add to your blender

Place chia seeds in a coffee grinder and chop to powder, brush the powder into your blender

Pit the cherries and add them to your blender

Wash and dry the spinach and chop

Add to the mix

Cover and blend on low followed by medium

Taste the texture and serve chilled!

The Sunshine Offering

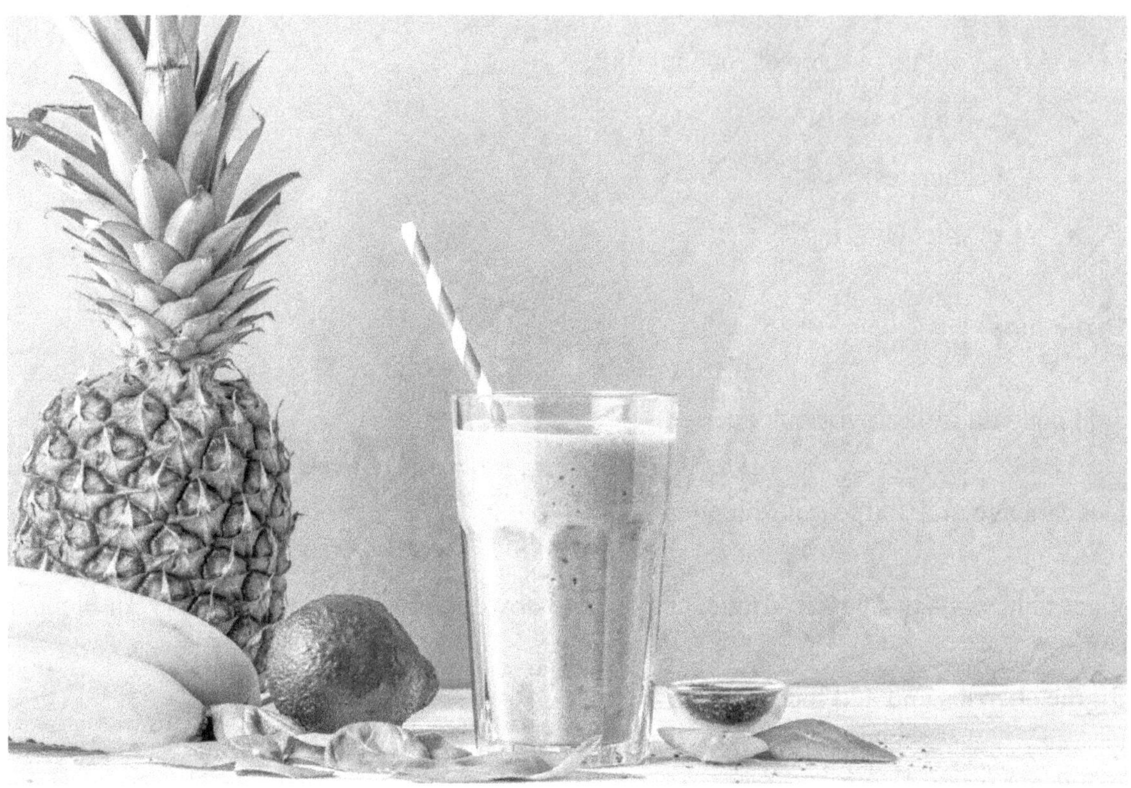

The Sunshine Offering Smoothie is a blend that tastes delicious and contains many antioxidants.

Servings: 2

Cook Time: 5 minutes

Ingredients

- 2 c. fresh spinach
- 1½ c. almond milk
- ½ c. coconut water
- 3 c. fresh pineapple
- 2 tbsp. coconut unsweetened flakes

Directions

Add all the listed ingredients to your blender

Blend until smooth

Add a few ice cubes and serve the smoothie

Enjoy!

The Sleepy Bug Smoothie

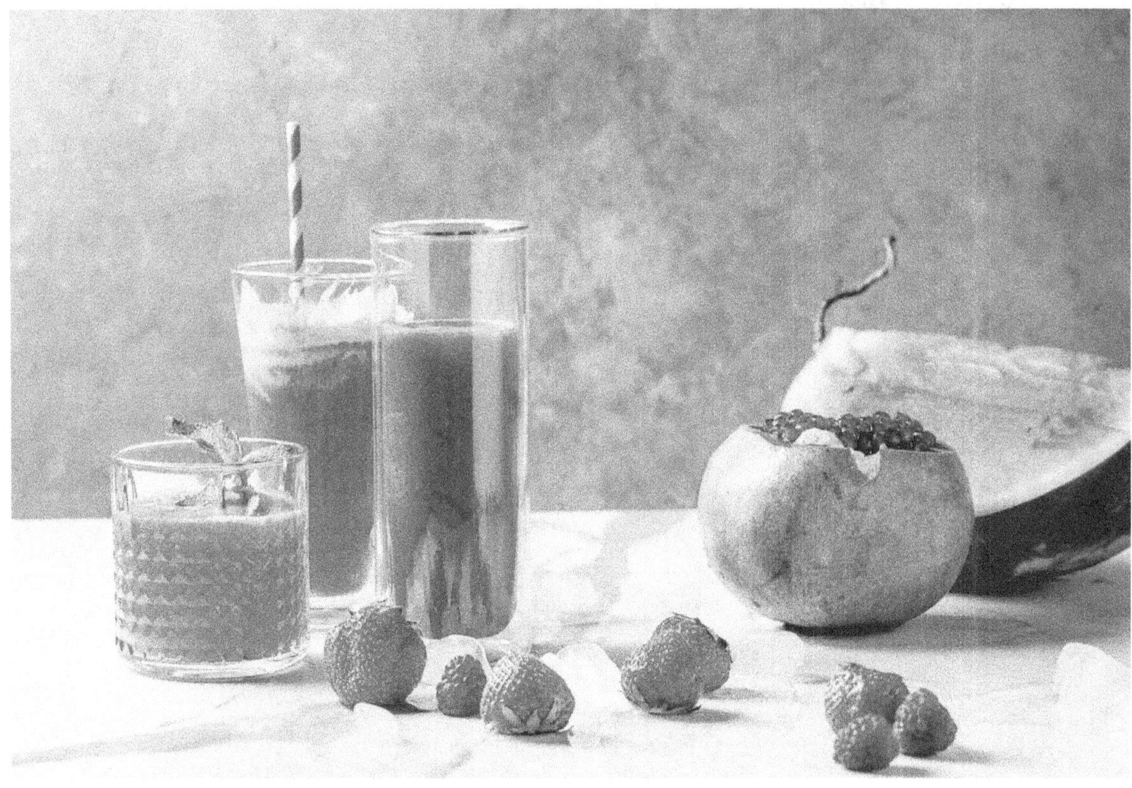

The Sleepy Bug Smoothie is a delicious treat that is helpful in healthy sleeping because of the natural sedative in it. It is a good way to enjoy a special treat and also helps you sleep better.

Servings: 2

Cook Time: 5 minutes

Ingredients

- 1 c. fennel tea infusion
- 1 c. almond milk
- 1 c. chopped watermelon
- 1 green apple
- ½ c. pomegranate
- ½ inch ginger
- Stevia to sweeten

Directions

Add the listed ingredients to your blender

Blend until smooth

Add a bit of stevia if you want more sweetness

Serve chilled and enjoy!

Matcha Coconut Smoothie

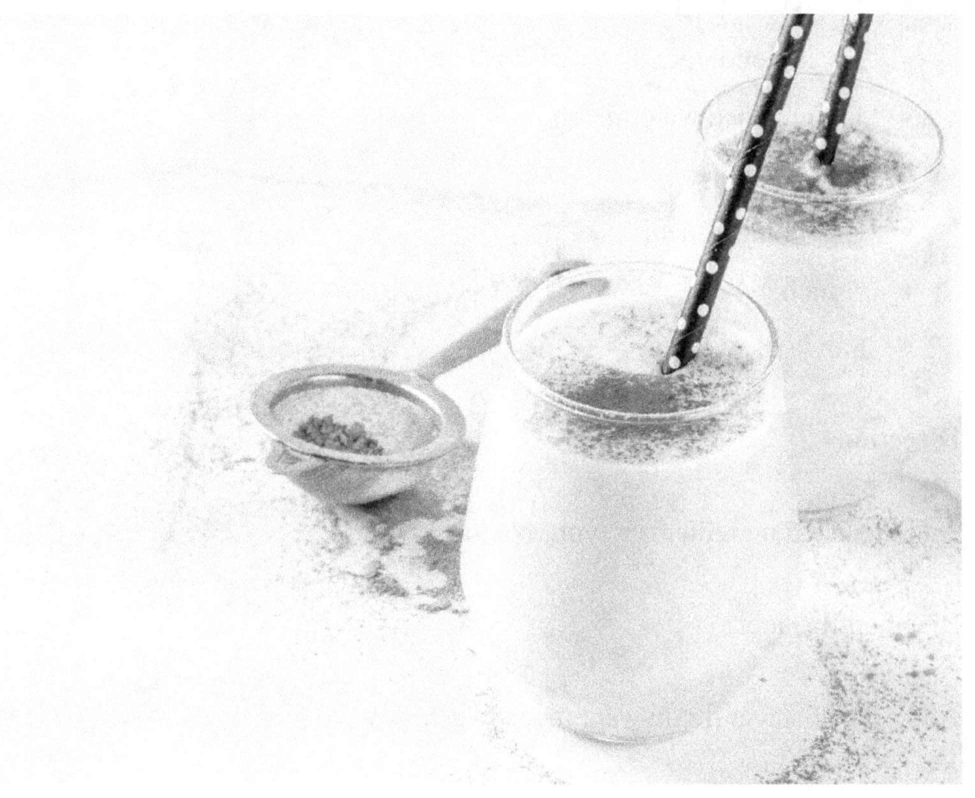

Matcha Coconut Smoothie is a great way to get your matcha fix while you are out and on the go. It is good to take with you on a morning walk or hike, or when you have to go out in the morning and want a healthy treat that is not sugary.

Servings: 2

Cook Time: 5 minutes

Ingredients

- 1 whole banana, cubed
- 1 c. frozen mango, chunked
- 2 kale leaves, torn
- 3 tbsp. white beans
- 2 tbsp. shredded coconut
- ½ tsp. matcha green tea powder
- 1 c. water

Directions

Add banana, kale, mango, matcha powder and white beans to your blender

Blend until you have a nice smoothie

Add shredded coconut as topping

Serve and enjoy!

Kale and Apple Smoothie

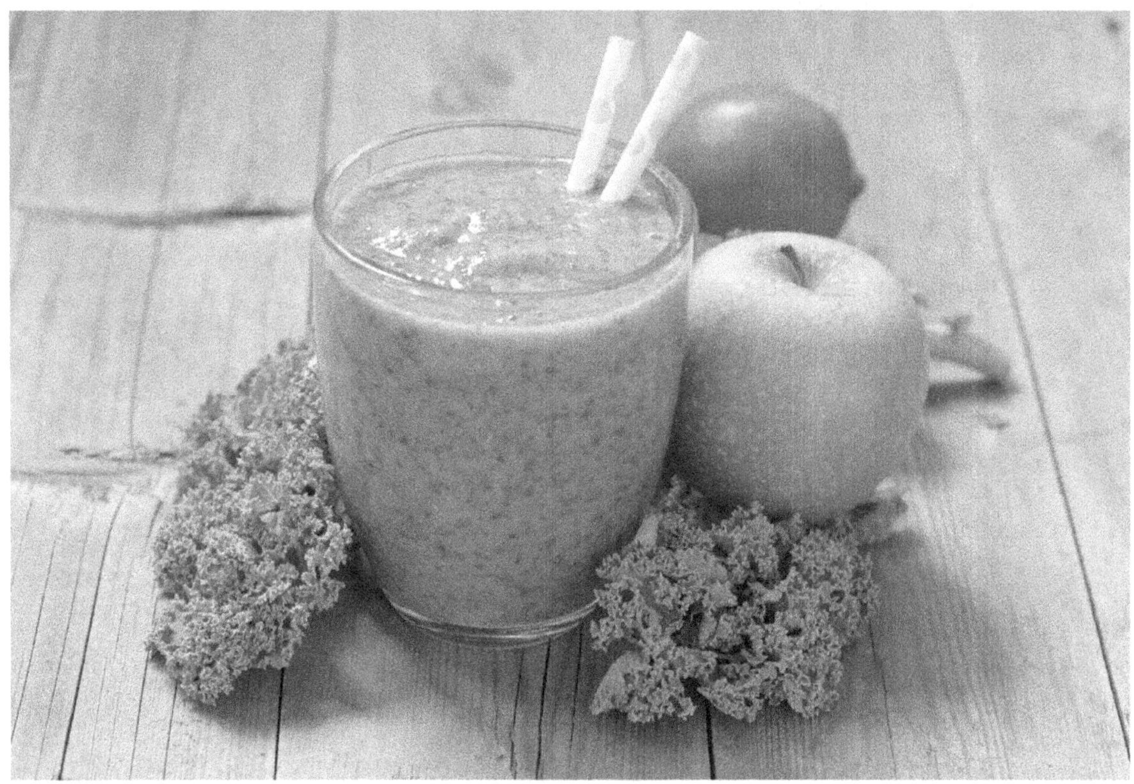

Kale and Apple Smoothie is a great healthy treat. It is good for everyone, especially kids. Starting the morning with these healthy drinks is a good idea. It is also a very good way to get some extra greens into your diet.

Servings: 2

Cook Time: 5 minutes

Ingredients

- ¾ of a kale, chopped, ribs and stem removed
- 1 small stalk celery, chopped
- ½ banana
- ½ c. apple juice
- 1 tbsp. lemon juice

Directions

Add the listed ingredients to your blender and blend until smooth

Serve chilled!

Beet & Strawberry Smoothie

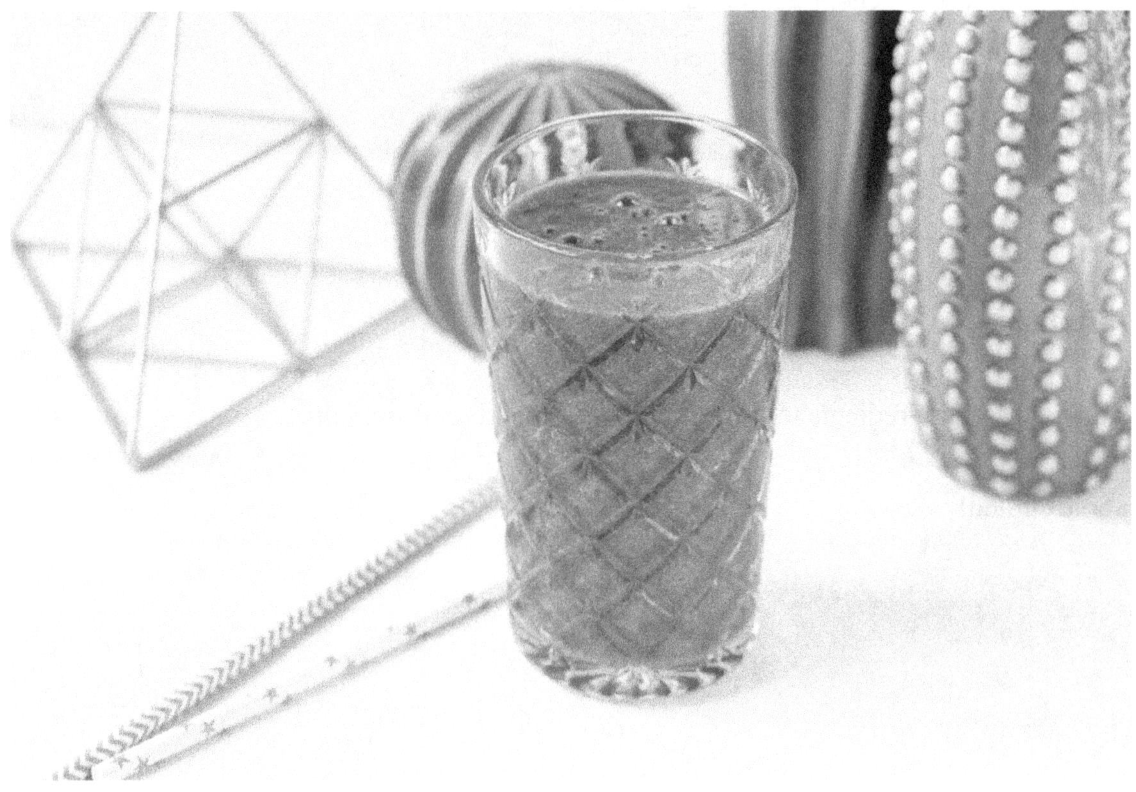

Beet & Strawberry Smoothie is a delicious drink perfect for everyone. It can be eaten at any time of year but is especially yummy in the summer.

Cook time: 10 minutes

Servings: 2

Ingredients:

- 2 c. frozen strawberries, pitted and chopped
- ⅔ roasted and frozen beet, chopped
- 1 tsp. fresh ginger, peeled and grated
- 1 tsp. fresh turmeric, peeled and grated
- ½ c. fresh orange juice
- 1 c. unsweetened almond milk

Directions

Place all the ingredients in a high-speed blender and pulse until creamy.

Pour the smoothie into two glasses and serve immediately.

Pineapple & Carrot Smoothie

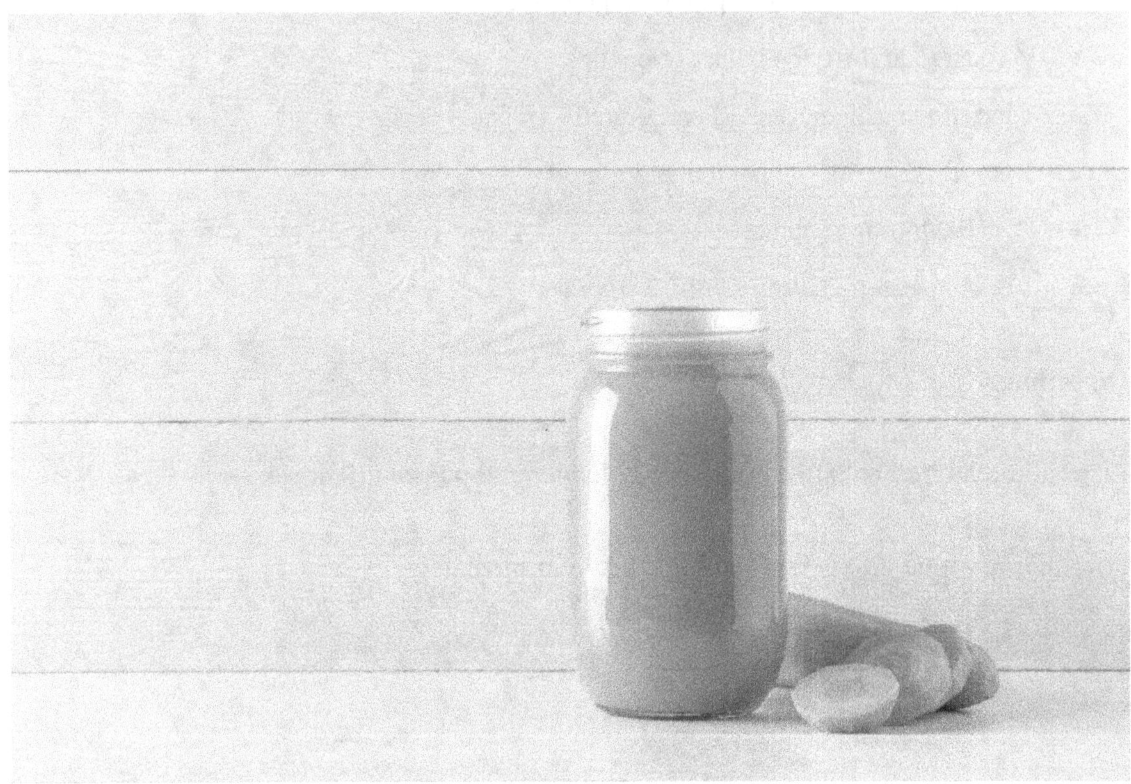

Pineapple & Carrot Smoothie is a tropical treat that is full of flavor. It is a nice way to start off your day. This smoothie is best made with fresh or frozen pineapple for maximum flavor.

Cook time: 10 minutes

Servings: 2

Ingredients:

- 1 c. frozen pineapple
- 1 ripe banana, peeled and sliced
- ½ tbsp. fresh ginger, peeled and chopped
- ¼ tsp. ground turmeric
- 1 c. unsweetened almond milk
- ½ c. fresh carrot juice
- 1 tbsp. fresh lemon juice

Directions

Place all the ingredients in a high-speed blender and pulse until creamy.

Pour the smoothie into two glasses and serve immediately.

Coconut Macaroon Smoothie

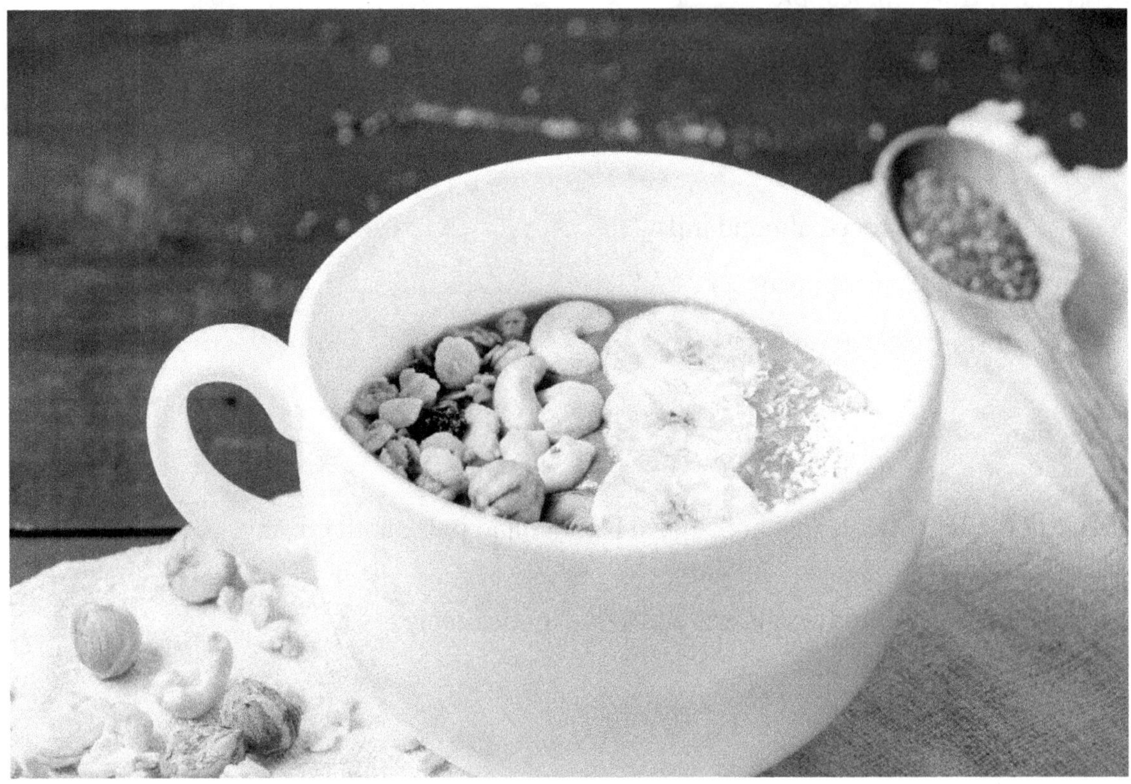

Coconut Macaroon Smoothie is a scrumptious nutritious that is blended with the taste of luxurious macaroons. It has all the benefits of coconut milk, but with a delightful smoothie flavor, this is a perfectly balanced beverage, excellent for your health.

Cook time: 6 minutes

Servings: 2

Ingredients

- 1 (14 oz.) can coconut milk
- 1 tsp. vanilla extract
- ½ c. cooked quinoa
- ¼ c. shredded coconut, unsweetened
- 2 Medjool dates, pitted and halved
- 1 c. ice cubes

Directions

Add everything in a blender and blend for 1 minute.

Cranberry-Orange Smoothie

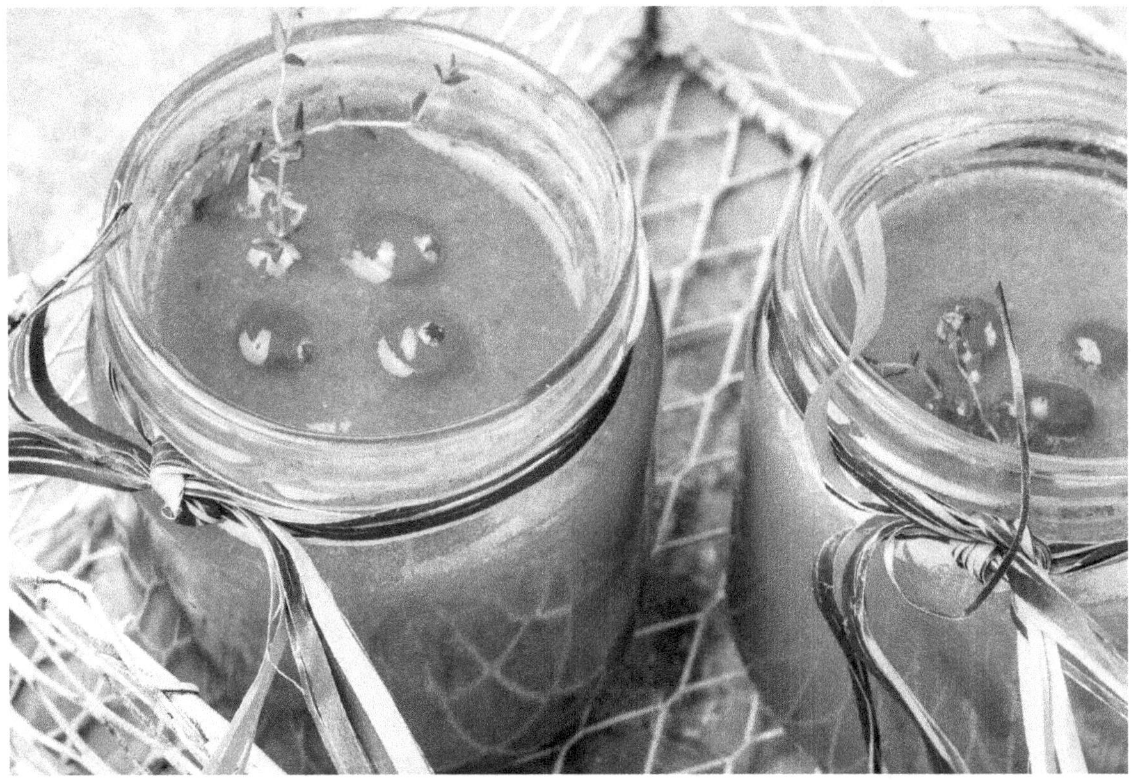

Cranberry-Orange Smoothie is a yummy blend to enjoy during the fall and winter months. It is a blend that is full of delicious flavor and has so much to offer the body and mind. It has some wonderful antioxidants and is a great smoothie to enjoy during the fall.

Cook time: 6 minutes

Servings: 2

Ingredients

- 2 oranges, rinds washed
- ½ c. alkaline water
- ½ avocado, pitted and halved
- 1 c. frozen cranberries
- 1 c. ice cubes

Directions

Cut the oranges into quarters and remove the rinds. Set 2 pieces of rind aside.

Blender everything in a blender for 1 minute.

Desserts and Snacks

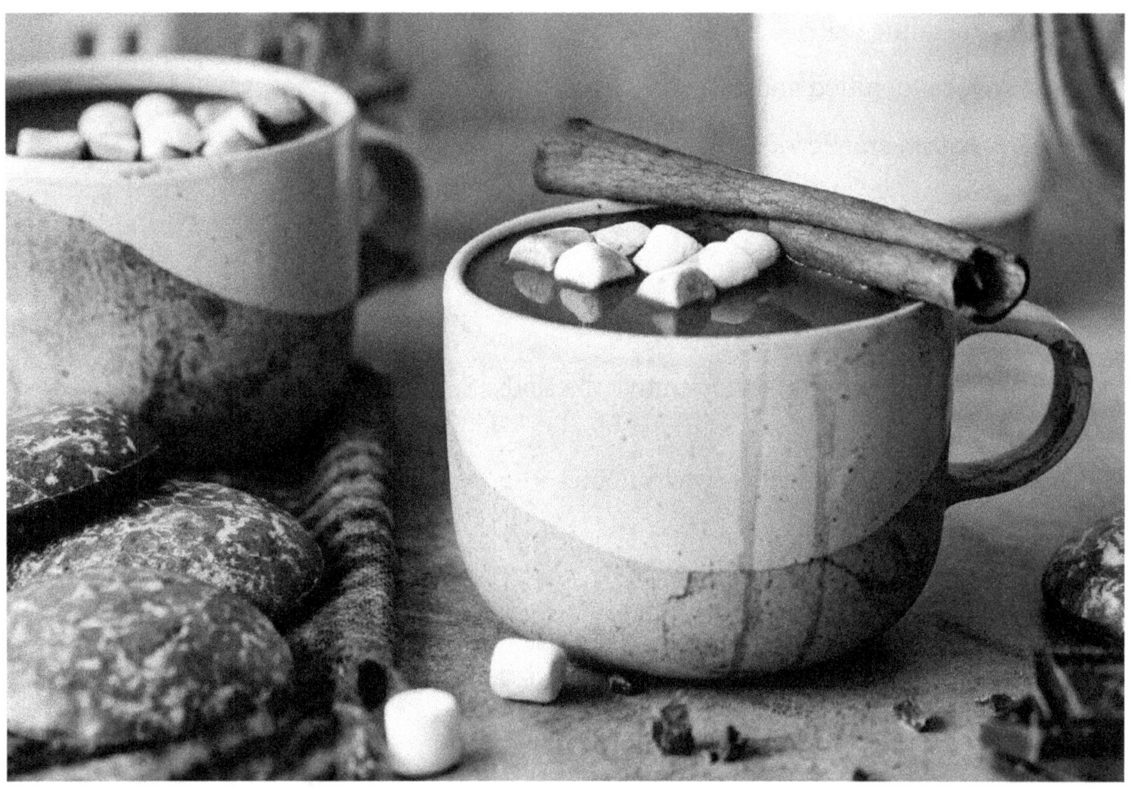

Alkaline Desserts and Snacks Recipes are very healthy for your heart, immune system, bones, skin, and brain. And, it is very easy to make. The ingredients are simply the best for you. And the good thing is that you can make it at your home. You can use any fruit you like, such as bananas, pineapple, apples, peaches, watermelon, pears, oranges, grapes, kiwi, papaya, coconut, strawberries, and mango. But to be ANTI-AGING, you have to use the right recipes. For example, beet is very healthy. But, just to add color to your dessert, it may not be a good idea to have a sugary dessert.

Mixed Berry Granita

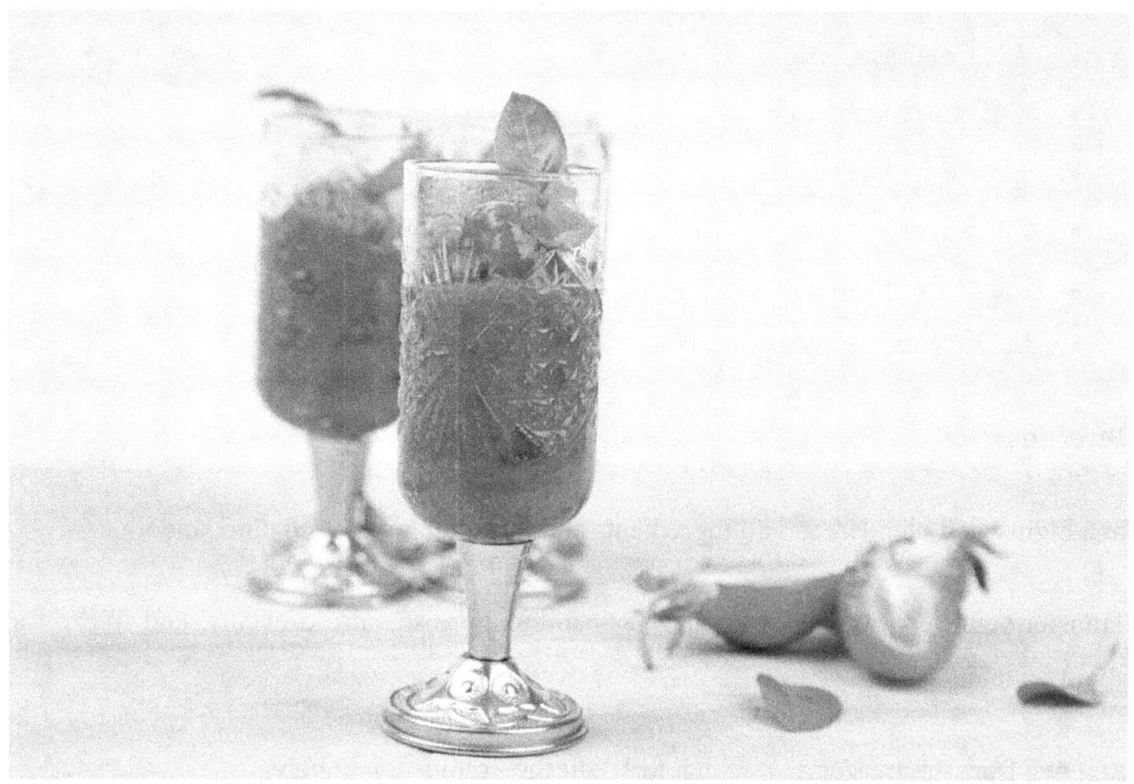

Mixed Berry Granita is a quick, easy, and deliciously healthy recipe that can be made with any berries.

Cook time: 15 minutes

Servings: 4

Ingredients:

- ½ c. fresh strawberries, hulled and sliced
- ½ c. fresh raspberries
- ½ c. fresh blueberries
- ½ c. fresh blackberries
- 1 tbsp. maple syrup
- 1 tbsp. fresh lemon juice
- 1 c. ice cubes, crushed

Directions

In a high-speed blender, add all ingredients and pulse on high speed until smooth.

Transfer your berry mixture into an 8x8-inch baking dish, spread evenly, and freeze for about 30 minutes.

Remove from the freezer and, with a fork, stir the granita completely.

Freeze for 2-3 hours, stirring every 30 minutes with a fork.

Strawberry Ice Cream

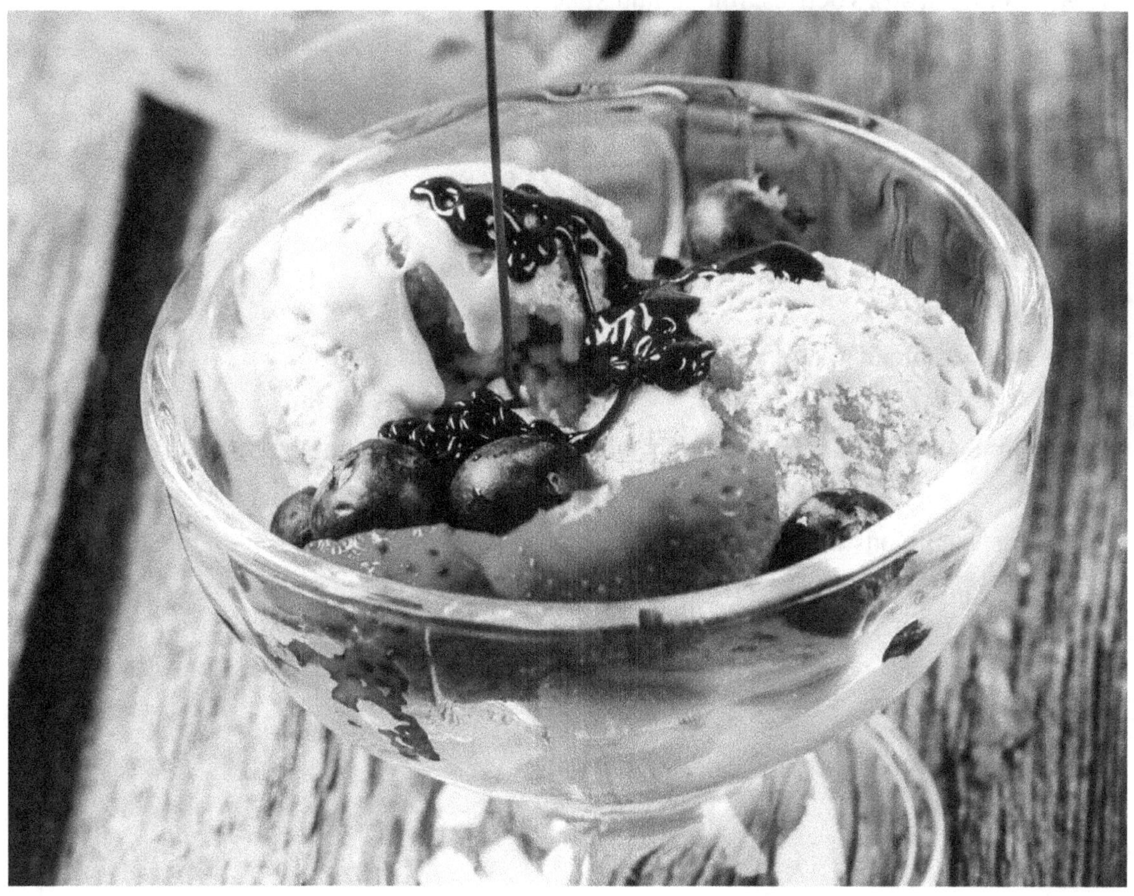

Strawberry Ice Cream is a fresh and delicious recipe for any time of the year! There are many ways to make ice cream in a healthy way. This recipe is perfect for someone who wants to stay away from foods that are high in sugar. This recipe is also a great way of using your fresh fruit that may be left over after you make other treats.

Cook time: 15 minutes

Servings: 4

Ingredients:

- 1 c. fresh strawberries, hulled and sliced
- ½ small banana, peeled and sliced
- 2 tbsp. coconut, shredded
- ½ c. coconut cream

Directions

In a high-speed blender, add all ingredients and pulse until smooth.

Transfer into an ice cream maker and process according to manufacturer's directions.

Now, transfer into an airtight container and freeze to set for at least 3-4 hours, stirring after every 30 minutes.

Hot Coconut Chocolate

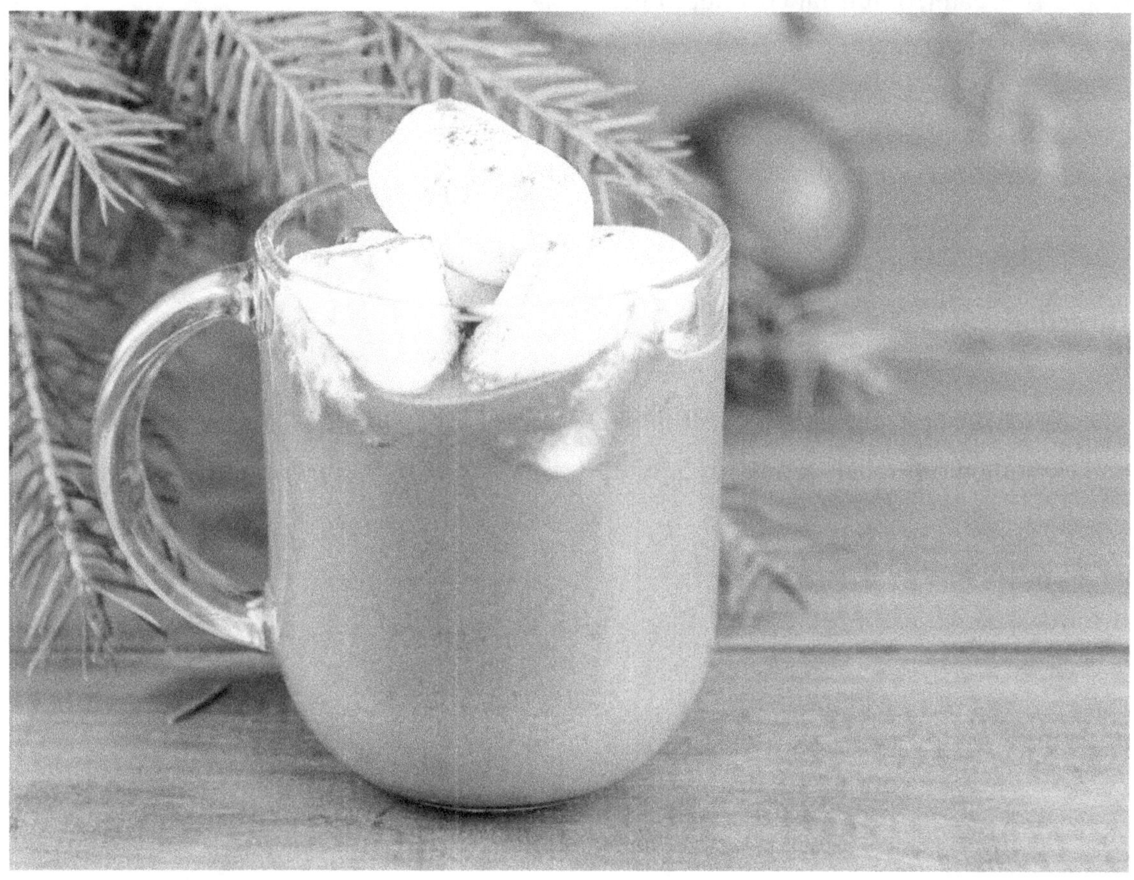

Hot Coconut Chocolate is a deliciously warm, rich chocolate drink that tastes wonderful for your winter nights! You can also make it with other great natural ingredients to include fall flavors such as cinnamon, ginger, and other spices.

Cook time: 5 minutes

Servings: 4

Ingredients

- 1 c. canned, full-fat coconut milk
- 1 c. filtered water
- 5 tbsp. cocoa powder
- 20 drops of liquid stevia, plus more as needed
- Ground cinnamon, for sprinkling

Directions

In a saucepan over medium heat, combine the cocoa powder, coconut milk, water, stevia, and cinnamon (optional). Cook for 5 minutes. Make sure no lump remains.

Taste and adjust seasoning.

Blueberry-Ginger Pudding

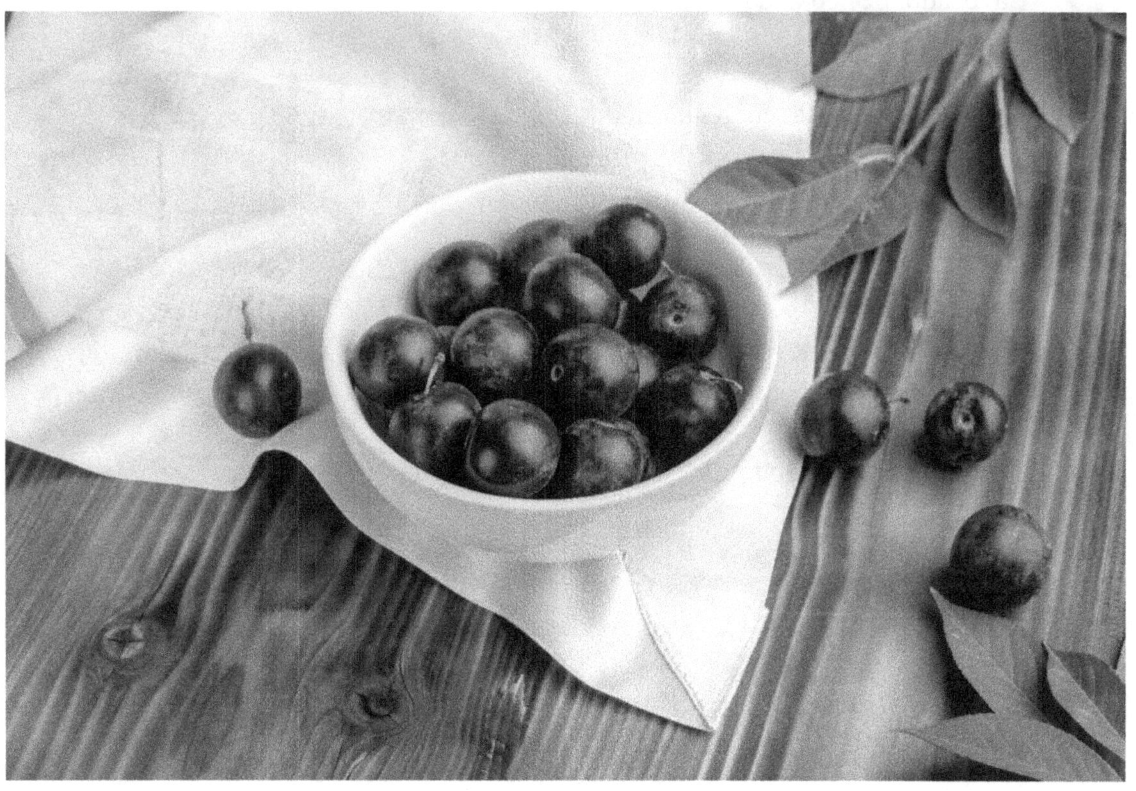

Blueberry-Ginger Pudding is a wonderful dessert that is easy to make and a great way to use fresh ingredients in your kitchen.

Cook time: 5 minutes

Servings: 2

Ingredients

- 1 avocado, peeled and pitted
- 1 c. frozen blueberries
- ¼ c. canned, full-fat coconut milk
- Juice of ½ lemon
- 1 tsp. fresh ginger, peeled and grated
- 10 drops liquid stevia

Directions

Combine everything in a food processor. Process until smooth.

Raspberry Jelly

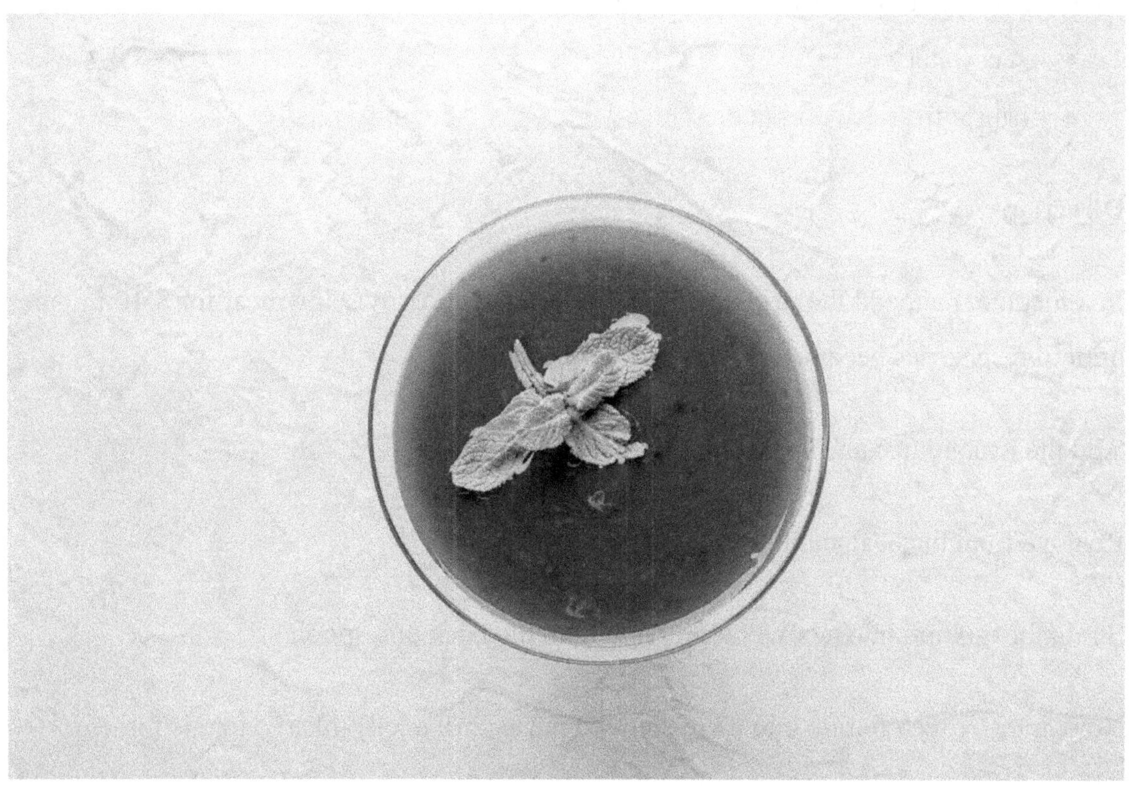

Raspberry Jelly is a great fruit snack for children and a great topping to a dessert. We have included some add-in ideas to make this jelly more interesting.

Cook time: 40 minutes

Servings: 4

Ingredients:

- 2 lb. fresh raspberries
- ¼ c. water
- 1 tbsp. fresh lemon juice

Directions

In a medium pan, add the raspberries and water and cook over low heat for 8-10 minutes or until raspberries become soft, stirring occasionally.

Add the lemon juice and cook for 30 minutes.

Remove from the heat and place the mixture into a sieve.

Strain the mixture into a bowl by pressing with the back of a spoon.

Now, transfer the mixture into a blender and pulse until a jelly-like texture is formed.

Transfer into glass serving bowls and refrigerate for at least 1 hour before serving.

Chickpea Fudge

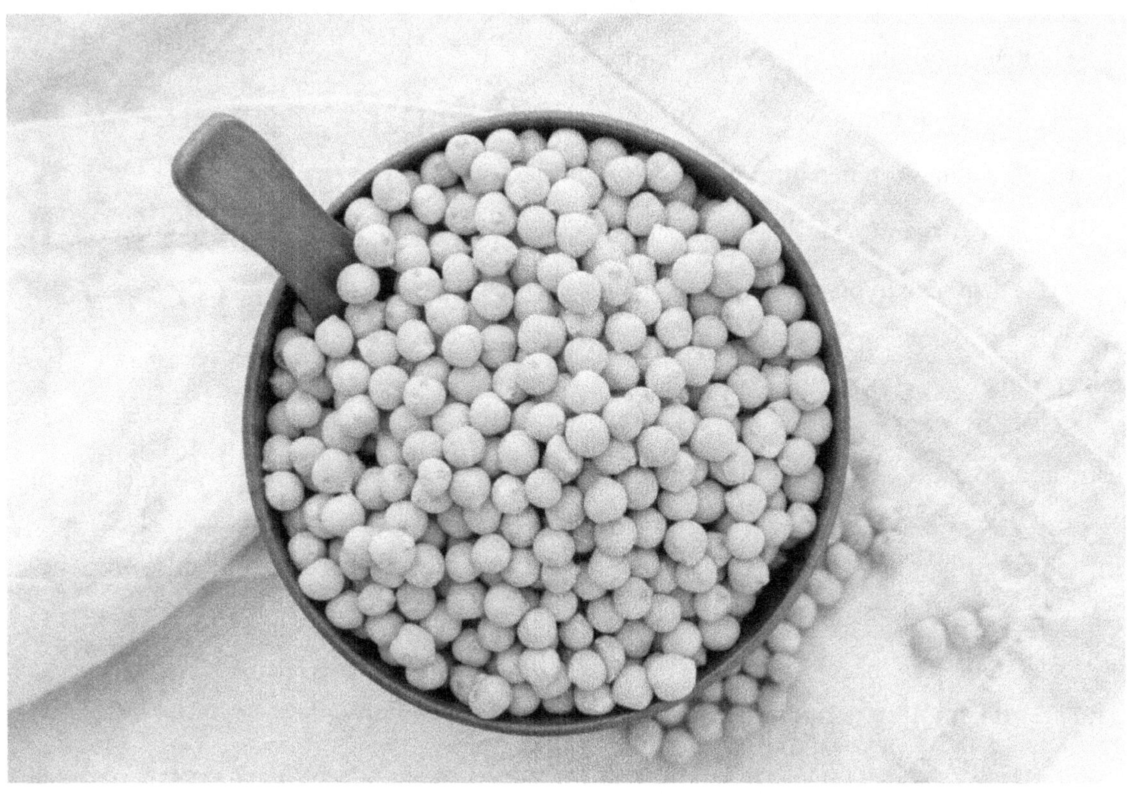

Chickpea Fudge Bars are a great way to use chickpeas. It is an easy snack that can be cut into different sized pieces.

Cook time: 15 minutes

Servings: 12

Ingredients:

- 2 c. cooked chickpeas
- 8 Medjool dates, pitted and chopped
- ½ c. almond butter
- ½ c. unsweetened almond milk
- 1 tsp. organic vanilla extract
- 2 tbsp. cacao powder

Directions

Line a large baking dish with parchment paper.

In a food processor, add all the ingredients except cacao powder and pulse until well combined.

Transfer the mixture into a large bowl and stir in the cacao powder.

Transfer the mixture into the prepared baking dish, evenly spread. Smooth the surface with the back of a spatula.

Refrigerate for about 2 hours or until set completely.

Cut into desired sized squares and serve.

Blackberry Crumble

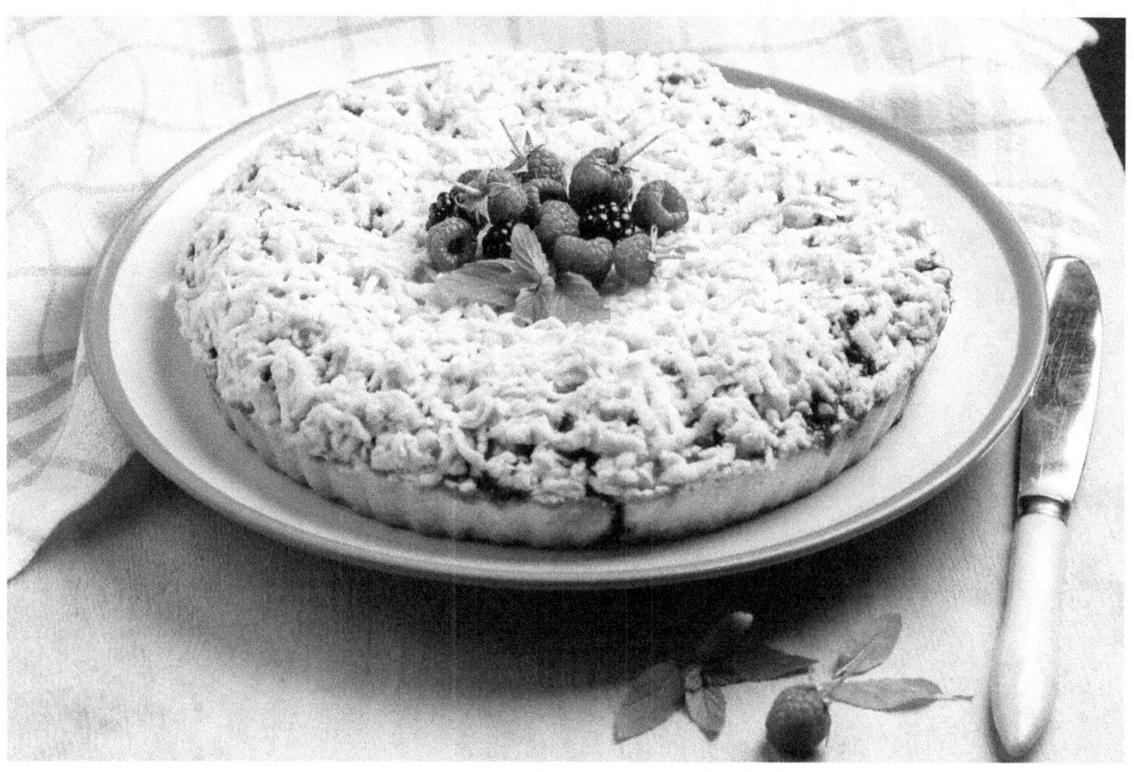

Blackberry Crumble is a delicious dessert that everyone will love.

Cook time: 50 minutes

Servings: 4

Ingredients:

- 1½ c. fresh blackberries
- 3 tbsp. water
- ½ tbsp. fresh lemon juice
- ¼ c. banana, peeled and mashed
- 2 tbsp. coconut oil, melted
- ¾ tsp. baking soda
- ¼ c. arrowroot flour
- ¼ c. coconut flour

Directions

Preheat the oven to 3oo degrees F. Lightly, grease an 8x8-inch baking dish.

In a large bowl, mix together all ingredients except blackberries.

Place blackberries in the bottom of prepared baking dish.

Spread flour mixture over blackberries evenly.

Bake for 35-40 minutes or until top becomes golden brown.

Serve warm.

No-Bake Cheesecake

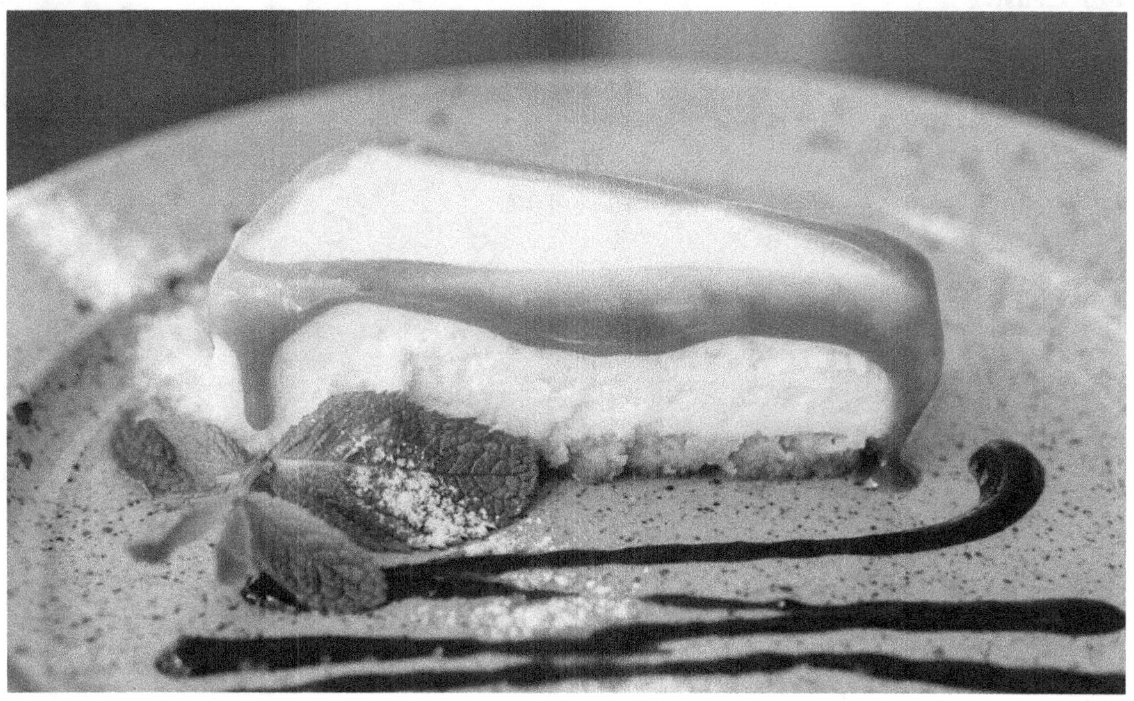

No-Bake Cheesecake recipe is easy to make and so delicious! It is one of our favorite recipes using cashews.

Cook time: 20 minutes

Servings: 12

Ingredients:

For Crust:

- 1 c. dates, pitted and chopped
- 1 c. raw almonds
- 3 tbsp. unsweetened coconut, shredded

For Filling:

- 3½ c. cashews, soaked overnight
- ½ c. coconut oil, melted
- 2 tbsps. fresh lemon rind, grated finely
- ¾ c. fresh lemon juice
- ¾ c. maple syrup
- 10 drops liquid stevia
- 1 tsp. vanilla extract
- Salt, to taste

Directions

For the crust: in a food processor, add the dates, almonds, and coconut and pulse until mixture just starts to combine.

Transfer the mixture into a greased springform pan and, with the back of a spatula, smooth the surface of the crust.

For the filling: in the clean food processor, add the cashews and oil and pulse until well combined.

Add the remaining ingredients, except lemon slices and pulse until creamy and smooth.

Pour the mixture over crust evenly and with the back of a spatula, smooth the top.

Refrigerate for about 1 hour.

Cut into 12 equal-sized slices and serve.

Strawberry Gazpacho

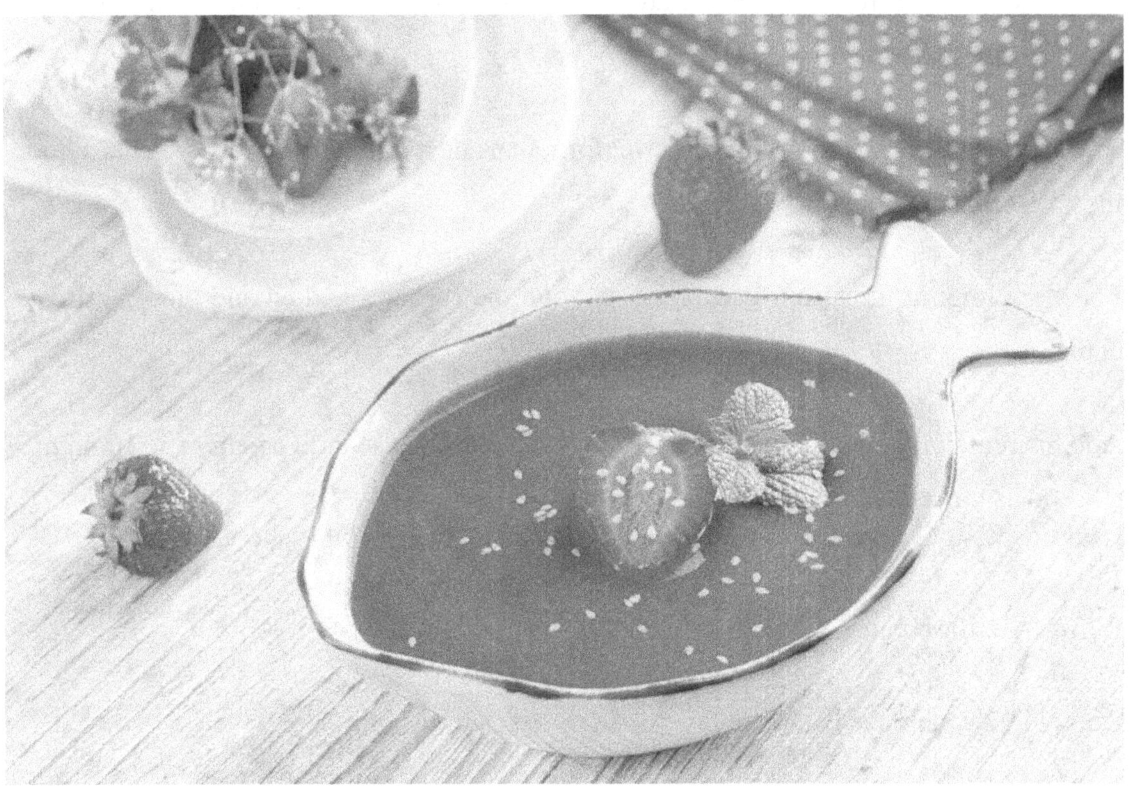

Strawberry Gazpacho is a refreshing and delicious soup. We use vinegar for this recipe because it has amazing health benefits.

Cook time: 15 minutes

Servings: 4

Ingredients:

- 1½ lb. fresh strawberries, hulled and sliced, plus extra for garnishing
- ½ c. red bell pepper, seeded and chopped
- 1 small cucumber, peeled, seeded, and chopped
- ¼ c. onion, chopped
- ¼ c. fresh basil leaves
- 1 small garlic clove, chopped
- ¼ small jalapeño pepper, seeded and chopped
- 1 tbsp. olive oil
- 2 tbsp. apple cider vinegar

Directions

In a high-speed blender, add 1½ lbs. of the strawberries and remaining ingredients and pulse until well combined and smooth.

Transfer the gazpacho into a large serving bowl.

Cover the bowl and refrigerate for about 4 hours before serving.

Serve chilled with a garnish of strawberry slices.

Tomato Salsa

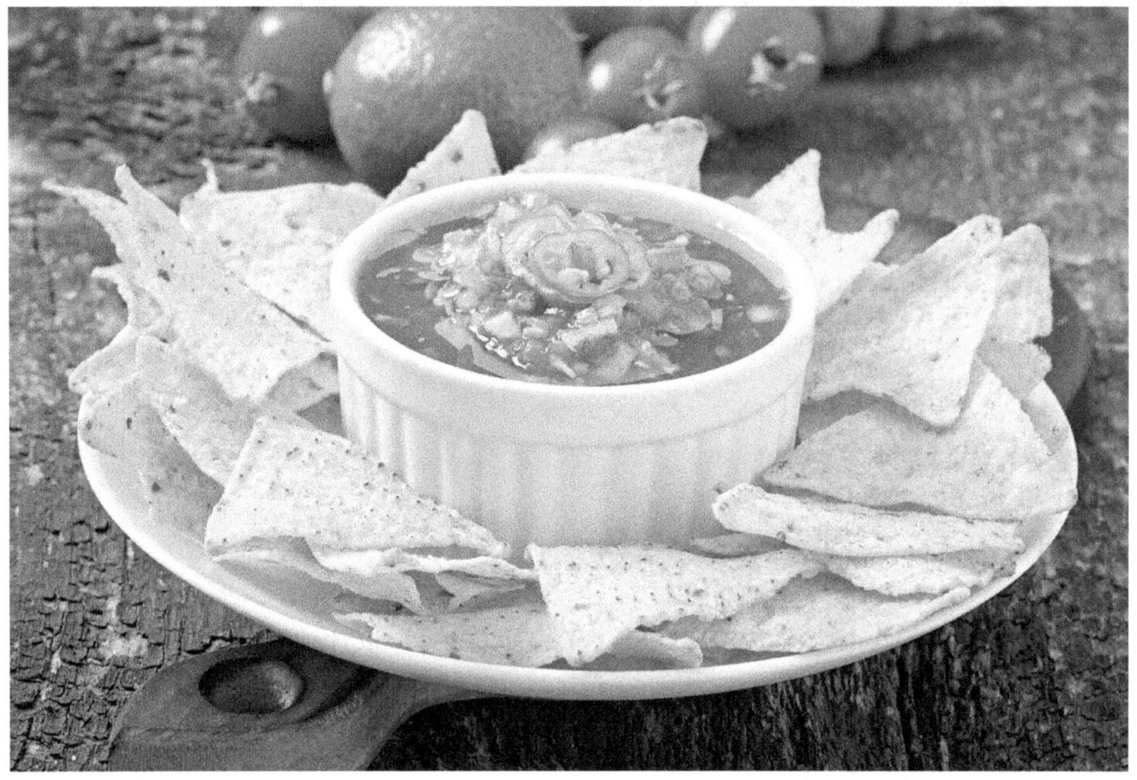

Tomato Salsa recipe is a quick and easy recipe that everyone will enjoy and love it!

Cook time: 10 minutes

Servings: 4

Ingredients:

- 3 large tomatoes, chopped
- 1 small red onion, chopped
- ¼ c. fresh cilantro leaves, chopped
- 1 jalapeño pepper, seeded and finely chopped
- 1 finely minced garlic clove
- 2 tbsp. fresh lime juice
- 1 tbsp. olive oil, extra-virgin
- Sea salt and ground black pepper

Directions

In a large bowl, add all the above ingredients and gently toss to coat well.

Serve immediately.

Avocado Guacamole

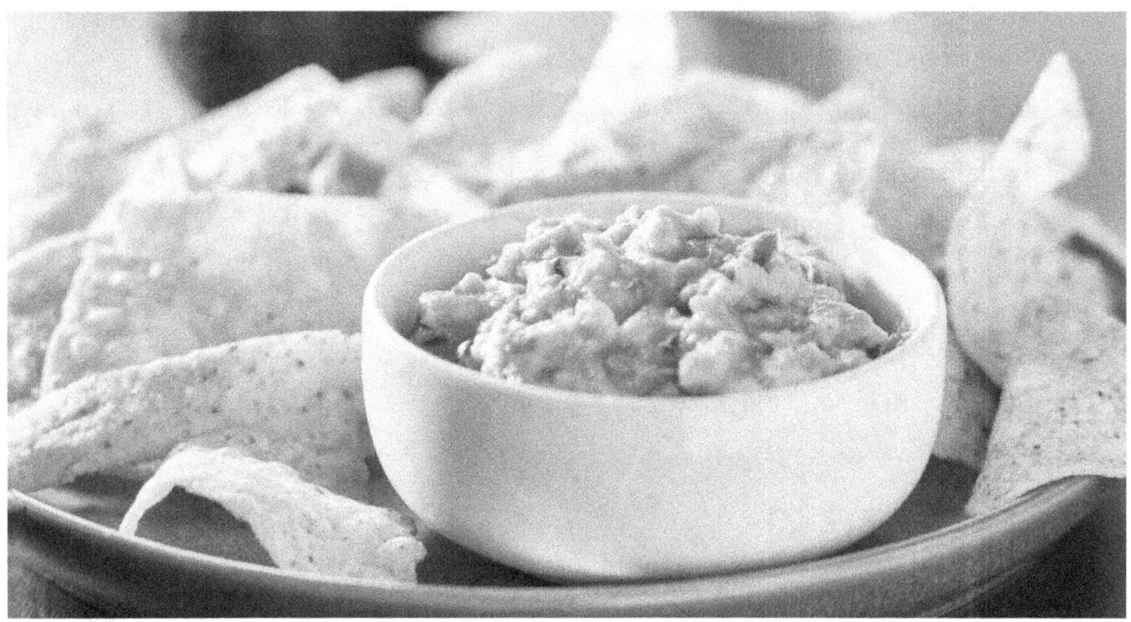

This simple avocado guacamole is perfect for dipping. Let's try it!

Cook time: 10 minutes

Servings: 4

Ingredients:

- 2 peeled and pitted ripe avocados, chopped
- 1 small chopped red onion
- 1 garlic clove, minced
- 1 seeded Serrano pepper, chopped
- 1 tomato, seeded and chopped
- 2 tbsp. fresh cilantro leaves, chopped
- 1 tbsp. fresh lime juice
- Salt, to taste

Directions

In a large bowl, add avocado and mash it completely with a fork.

Add the remaining ingredients and gently stir to combine.

Serve immediately.

Cauliflower Hummus

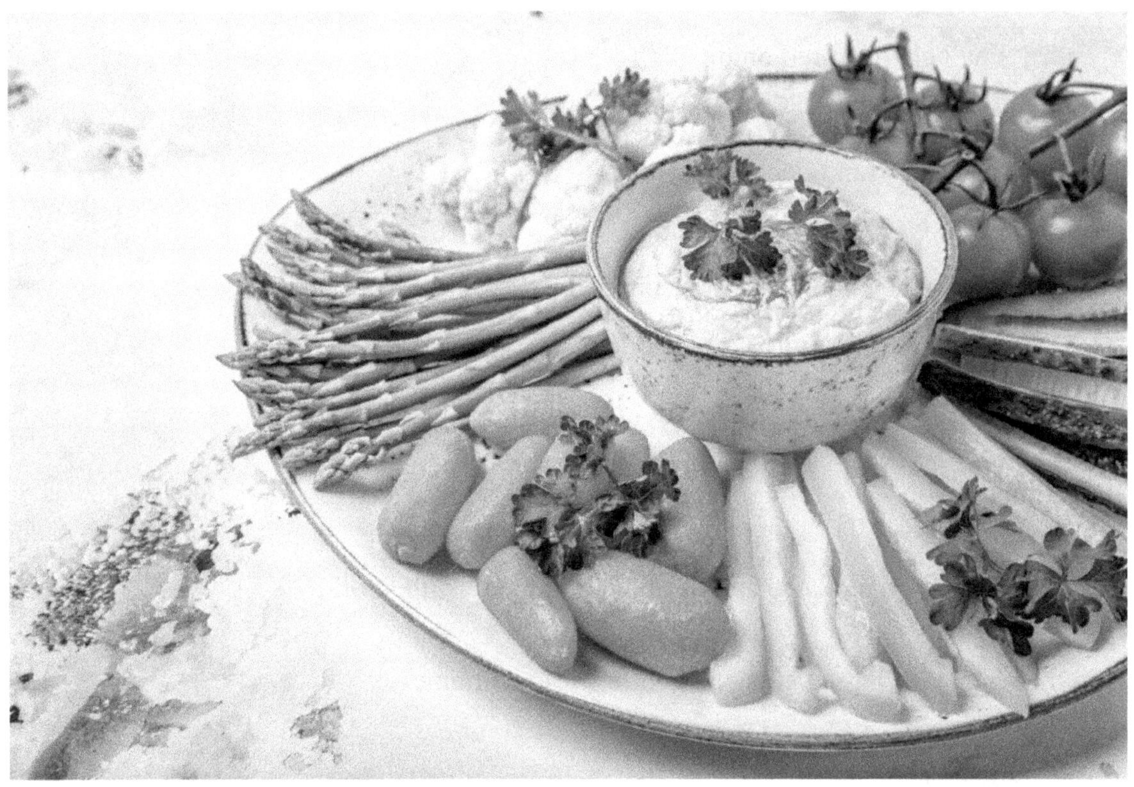

Got bored of the regular hummus? Try my healthy version of this appetizer with cauliflower! You will like it.

Cook time: 20 minutes

Servings: 6

Ingredients:

- 1 medium head cauliflower, trimmed and chopped
- 2 garlic cloves, chopped
- 2 tbsp. almond butter
- 2 tbsp. olive oil
- Salt, to taste
- 2 tbsp. fresh chives, minced
- Pinch of cayenne pepper

Directions

In a large pan of boiling water, add the cauliflower and reduce to medium heat. Cook for 4-5 minutes.

Remove from the heat and drain the cauliflower well.

Set aside to cool slightly.

In a food processor, add the cauliflower, garlic, almond butter, oil, and salt and pulse until smooth.

Transfer the hummus into a serving bowl.

Sprinkle with chives and cayenne pepper and serve immediately.

Devilled Eggs

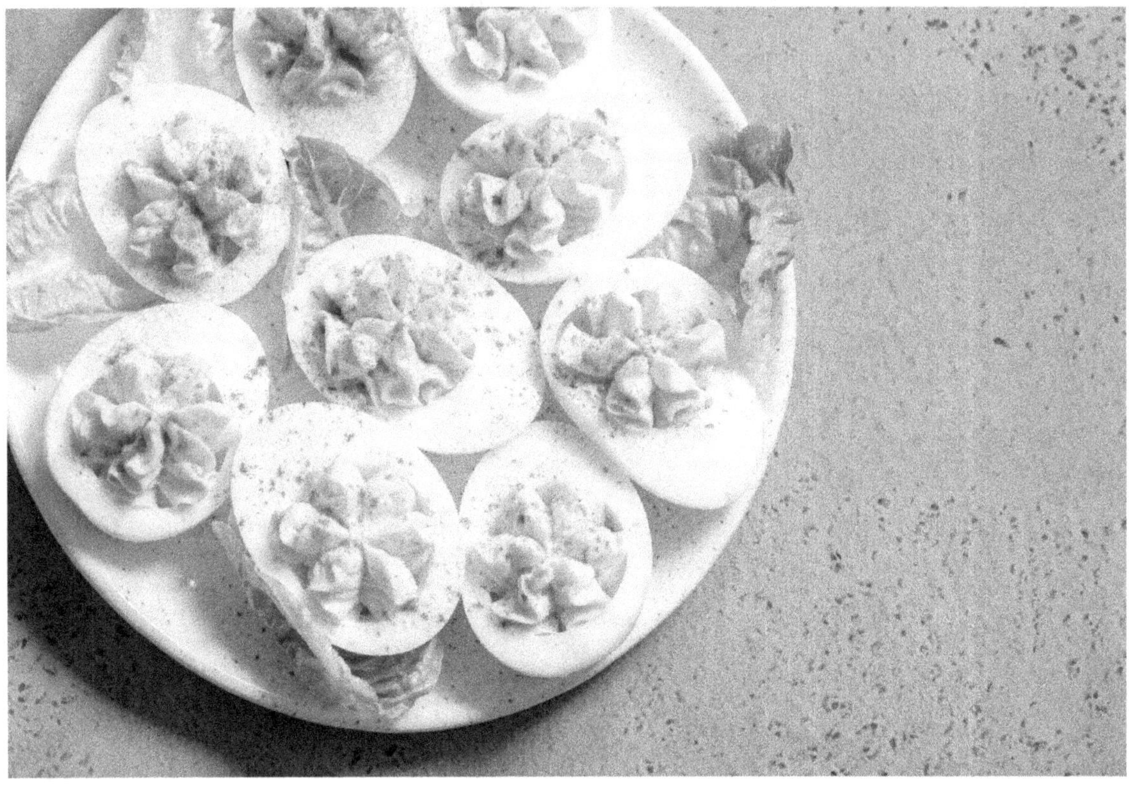

Devilled Eggs are an excellent snack food that many people enjoy. They are a great way to use up leftover herbs from other recipes.

Cook time: 15 minutes

Servings: 6

Ingredients:

- 6 large organic eggs
- 1 medium avocado, peeled, pitted, and chopped
- 2 tsp. fresh lime juice
- Sea salt, to taste
- Pinch of cayenne pepper

Directions

In a large pan of water, add the eggs and bring to a boil over high heat.

Cover the pan and immediately remove from the heat.

Set aside, covered for at least 10-15 minutes.

Drain the eggs and let them cool completely.

Peel the eggs and, with a sharp knife, slice them in half vertically.

Remove the yolks from egg halves.

In a bowl, add half of the egg yolks, avocado, lime juice, and salt and, with a fork, mash until well combined.

Scoop the avocado mixture into the egg halves evenly.

Serve with a sprinkling of cayenne pepper.

Wheat Crackers

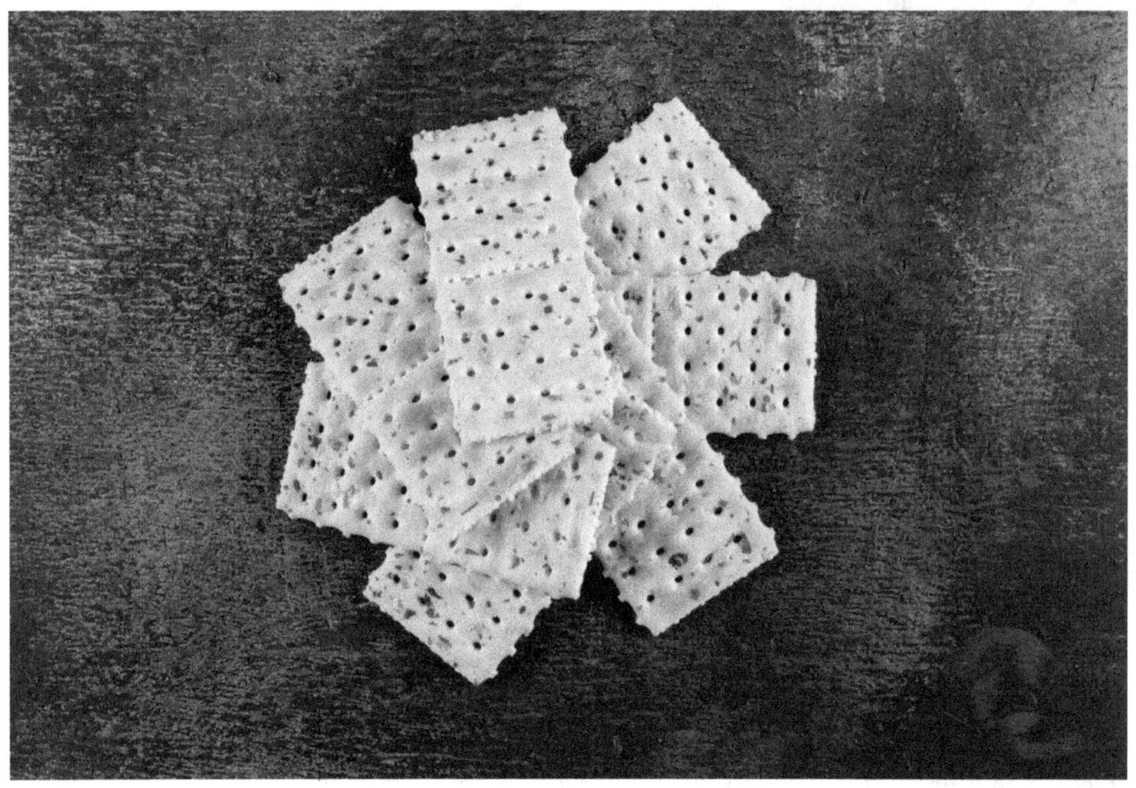

Wheat Crackers, a simple recipe for you when you want something new and different.

Cook time: 30 minutes

Servings: 4

Ingredients:

- 1¾ c. almond flour
- 1½ c. coconut flour
- ¾ tsp. sea salt
- 1/3 c. vegetable oil
- 1 c. alkaline water
- Sea salt for sprinkling

Directions

Set your oven to 350 degrees F.

Mix coconut flour, almond flour and salt in a bowl.

Stir in vegetable oil and water. Mix well until smooth.

Spread this dough on a floured surface into a thin sheet.

Cut small squares out of this sheet.

Arrange the dough squares on a baking sheet lined with parchment paper.

Bake for 20 minutes until light golden in color.

Potato Chips

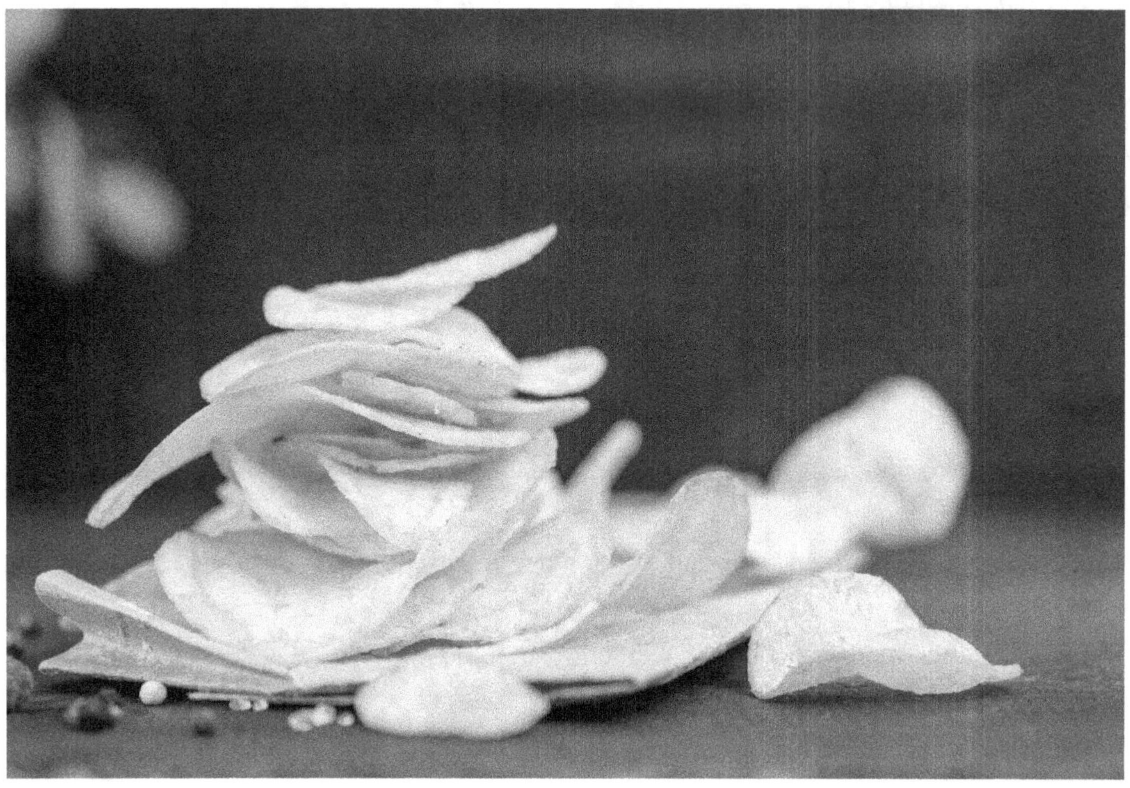

Potato Chips recipe is done right. They are easy to make, tasty, and a great snack. We have used fresh potatoes. We guarantee that you won't be disappointed!

Cook time: 10 minutes

Servings: 4

Ingredients:

- 1 tbsp. vegetable oil
- 1 potato, sliced paper thin
- Sea salt, to taste

Directions

Toss potato with oil and sea salt.

Spread the slices in a baking dish in a single layer.

Cook in a microwave for 5 minutes until golden brown.

Zucchini Pepper Chips

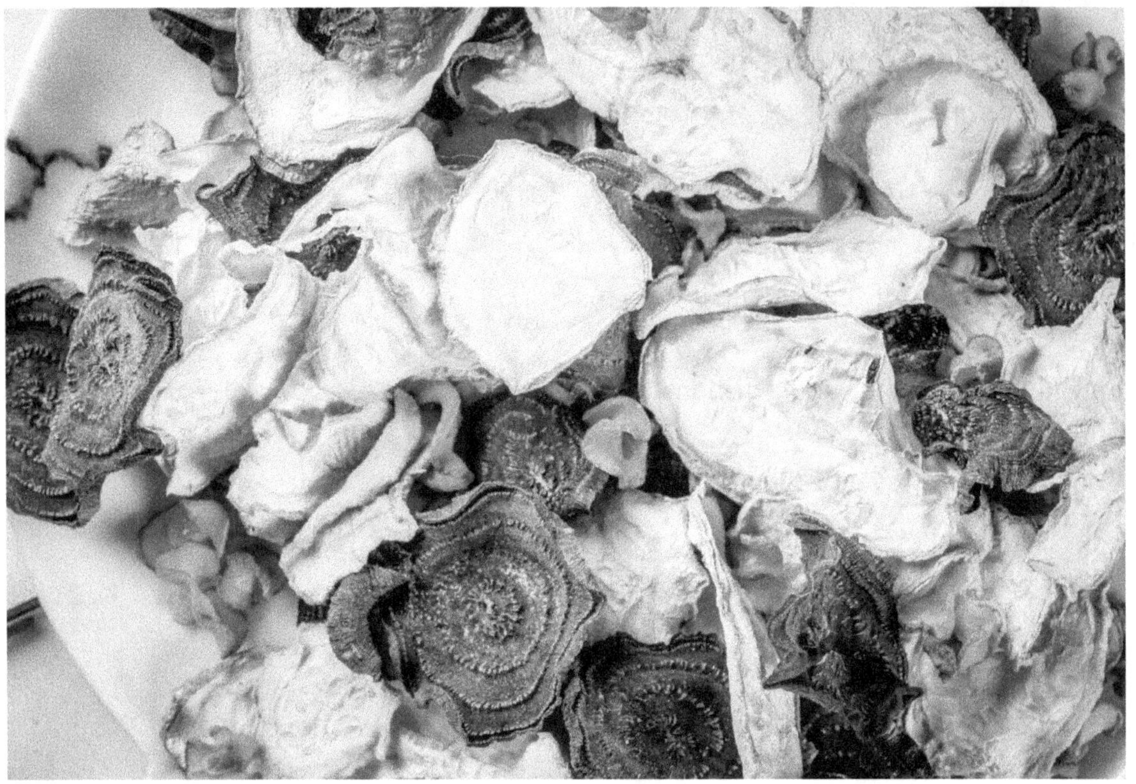

This recipe is easy to make and can be eaten at any time of the year. Enjoy!

Cook time: 25 minutes

Servings: 04

Ingredients:

- 1 2/3 c. vegetable oil
- 1 tsp. garlic powder
- 1 tsp. onion powder
- ½ tsp. black pepper
- 3 tbsp. crushed red pepper flakes
- 2 zucchinis, thinly sliced

Directions

Mix oil with all the spices in a bowl.

Add zucchini slices and mix well.

Transfer the mixture to a Ziplock bag and seal it.

Refrigerate for 10 minutes.

Spread the zucchini slices on a greased baking sheet.

Bake for 15 minutes

Conclusion

One of the biggest problems we're facing today is the low quality of food, as we're literally bombarded by processed foods and natural food is not accessible to everyone. Whether we're talking about restaurants or supermarkets, processed food is abundant. Around 70% of the diseases known today are caused by the food we eat, and we have to thank processed food for this. This type of food is very low in nutritional value and has all sorts of chemicals and added sugars that are harmful to your body. This is how we end up with high blood pressure, heart disease, type 2 diabetes, kidney stones, liver disease, or even more severe like cancer.

When it comes to processed food, everything is about profits, which basically means high quantity and low quality. Especially because of the mass-production techniques spawned by the philosophies of the Industrial Revolution, the poor quality of grains, fruits, and vegetables are accumulated in animals that eat those same poor agricultural products. Thus, the human diet consists of compounding layers of poor food quality.

The alkaline diet emphasizes balancing the pH level in your body. This indicator is the measurement unit for the ratio between the acid and alkaline levels in your body. Processed food has a very high acid level, and a high acid level leads to serious diseases. The purpose of the alkaline diet is to lower the acid level and increase the alkaline level in order to prevent such diseases and conditions. The alkaline diet encourages you to eat mostly veggies and fruits, which by default are more alkaline than acid.

Thank you and good luck!

Author's Afterthoughts

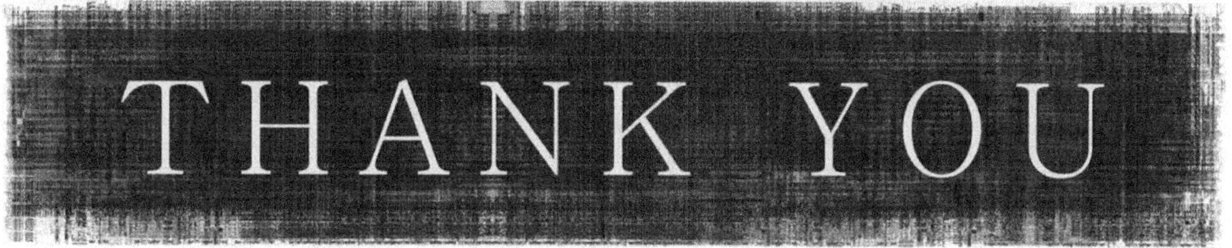

I am thankful for downloading this book and taking the time to read it. I know that you have learned a lot and you had a great time reading it. Writing books is the best way to share the skills I have with your and the best tips too.

I know that there are many books and choosing my book is amazing. I am thankful that you stopped and took time to decide. You made a great decision and I am sure that you enjoyed it.

I will be even happier if you provide honest feedback about my book. Feedbacks helped by growing and they still do. They help me to choose better content and new ideas. So, maybe your feedback can trigger an idea for my next book.

Thank you again

Sincerely

Ivy Hope